Rewilding COVID

Natural and Practical Health Solutions for Optimizing Your Immunity During the Coronavirus Pandemic and Beyond

JOHN SCHOTT

Publishing services provided by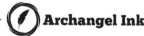

ISBN: 978-1-950043-26-2

STAY CONNECTED

Visit RewildingCovid.com to sign up for the latest news and natural health updates.

FOREWORD

We now live in a post-COVID world. That means that never before have health, wellness, and resilience been more important. The truth is, the state of one's "inner terrain" was always a life-and-death matter. The fact was just well hidden before COVID made everyone suddenly aware of its fundamental importance. But the conventional medical system would have us focus on gene defects and germs as the primary causes of what ails us.

We're coming into a time where many of us are beginning to see through this smokescreen. We're realizing that we are radically responsible for our own health—no victims are allowed to enter into the inner sanctum of this awareness. If we have co-created our illness, that implies that we have access to an immense power to uncreate it. Better yet, it implies we have the power to create immense health and vitality, if only we have the right tools.

This is why *Rewilding COVID* is such an exciting contribution. It is solutions-focused. It uses time-tested practices we can apply to take back full control of our health destinies. The COVID crisis, for me, reveals just how far humanity has strayed from nature and illuminates the natural principles we must follow to obtain and maintain perfect health. Hippocrates said it so well, "The natural healing force within each one of us is the greatest force in getting well."[1]

It takes a great shock to wake someone out of a deep stupor. COVID is that shock, and the structure and framework most needed to recover from that stupor will be laid down by books like this. We need to know what daily practices and principles will set us on the

---

1   "Hippocrates (460 BC–377 BC)," The Quotations Page, accessed October 19, 2020, http://www.quotationspage.com/quotes/Hippocrates/.

path to radical health sovereignty and a lived experience of strength, joy, and abundant health.

John, like many of us on this path, is both a wounded-healer and wounded-warrior who has figured out (with great effort and courage) how to alchemize the pain and suffering of wrong living (inherited by a sick society) into recovery, healing, and an even deeper strength that comes with overcoming life's great challenges. In sharing his stories and hard-won solutions, he's made it far easier for others to find their path to success and healing as well.

Let's all learn how to rewild ourselves and create the more beautiful world our hearts and minds know is possible, as my colleague Charles Eisenstein once said.

—Sayer Ji

CONTENTS

INTRODUCTION

It is quite clear that the COVID-19 phenomenon has shaken the foundations of our society. Whether you believe the predominant narrative or have been questioning the official story with skepticism and common sense, there is no doubt that we have all been affected.

Throughout the last few months, I have been observing the unfolding situation in silence. I've been analyzing perspectives, leaning into intuition, and relying on my deep connection to the web of life.

For most of my life I have been on a quest for knowledge and self-discovery. It's a path marked by looking beyond the mainstream narratives and messages of the mass media. I admit that I'm biased toward sovereignty and freedom. No matter what the current situation brings, I am in favor of empowerment, truth, and trust in the divine spirit of creation.

Many years ago I experienced the proverbial dark night of the soul. Fortunately, it was followed by the most powerful spiritual experience of my life. By then I had taken part in sacred ceremonies that included San Pedro and ayahuasca. I'd practiced extended fasting, meditation, and deep breathwork. But nothing I'd done compared to this. This was a moment that will live in my consciousness forever. It involved the spirit of God and an encounter with my grandfather who passed over twenty-four years ago. I woke at 4 a.m. in Long Island City, New York, to a majestic light flooding the room. This light was not natural to our plane of existence. I heard the voice of God clearly, and it asked me what I wanted. I wanted to hug my grandfather one more time since he had always been my hero and had left us way too early. I needed him more than ever in that moment.

1

This higher power answered, offering me the gift of my grandfather coming back to life and hugging me like only he could. He assured me everything was going to be fine, that my grandmother would be with him once again and would finally have eternal peace. As he left, the voice of God gave me the one answer I had always sought. It was simple. It didn't ask or require anything of me. He said all I needed to do was to simply love. The light slowly vanished, and I found myself back in the bed crying tears of deep joy, hope, and fulfillment.

My journey into the field of health and wellness has always been fueled by a desire to help humanity. After that life-altering moment with my grandfather, I was even more determined to use health and lifestyle teachings to help others on their path to living their best life. I have spent over twelve years studying, experimenting, and working with clients from all walks of life to slowly perfect the principles laid out in this book. I have studied with PhDs, clinicians, chefs, nutrition pioneers, and innovators. And I have developed a meticulous self-taught approach.

Through the years, I've been a coach, deep bodyworker, health food chef, and an entrepreneur driven by the intent to help others. The culmination of these events and experiences have led me to a grounded approach in standing up to an invisible enemy. Make no mistake, we are in a battle for freedom. First, it's time to stop the war machine. It's volatile and irresponsible, and it has a high potential of destroying our species. Second, we can no longer continue our spiritual bypassing. It's time for us to take conscious action—as individuals and as a collective.

Each of us has a purpose. Whatever our calling, we can be driven by peace, justice, and equality. It is not my intention to make this work political; we have to go beyond that. There is no government, corporation, guru, or alternative Q movement coming to save us. Handing over our sovereignty to any external authority will lead us back to forced servitude and dependence.

The intention of this book is twofold:

1. To create awareness. A healthy level of skepticism is needed if we are to question common beliefs and discover a new paradigm.

2. To offer time-tested, context-based foundational practices that enhance natural immunity and build truly healthy humans. The key to our freedom (of speech, choice, movement, and thought) lies in self-accountability and a deep commitment to ourselves, our family, our community, and the higher force that created all of us. This will lead to a true living example of mind, body, and spiritual integration.

This book aims to remind us of the basics: what we need to fuel the human body and the natural processes that have made us a thriving organism of the earth for generations. These are natural and innate to our species. We don't need a novel solution; we need to return to nature's design in a way that fits our current era. After all, this is no longer the world of our ancestors.

Our predecessors did not have to face the extreme challenge of a global chemical industry, which has left modern human health in crisis. The presence of pesticides, herbicides, GMOs, acid rain, and pollution (like cyanide poisoning specific to COVID) has epigenetically altered the environment to such a degree that we must actively adapt to these changes. Artificial electromagnetic frequencies are also new to modern human experience and cause dramatic changes to our environment. Our sedentary lifestyles lead us to be disconnected from others. Our bare feet seldom touch the earth. Chronic stress runs rampant. All of these factors and more have irreparably changed our environment. We face the task of adapting to this new world.

Also, as we consider a so-called new threat that is upon us—whether that be COVID, riots, or even fear—we must face it head on if we are to dismantle it. There is no hiding from the challenges of this time. Ironically, this is a beautiful realization—it means that we have all the tools we need to overcome. We can take this unique opportunity to transcend any and all previous paradigms.

Although this book focuses on building natural immunity and is titled *Rewilding COVID*, the message is bigger than that. Ultimately, this book represents a commonsense action plan for self-empowerment.

This moment is a point of no return. We are being called to move away from the outdated model in which we take without giving back. It's a system fueled by selfish practice. It does not consider regeneration. It has forgotten the dynamic livelihood of all ecosystems present in our diverse environments. We are on the cusp of a modern-day collective upgrade. We are seeing a subtle movement drawing humans to connect to each other, to form bonds that will allow us to supersede all previous evolutionary paths. It's exciting. It's challenging. It is a necessary shift that will push us out of our comfort zone. But, in the end, it will result in massive growth.

The intention behind *Rewilding COVID* is simple but profound. We have to do more than merely overcome COVID. We can emerge once again as the dominant species, but one that functions with higher consciousness. We can finally become the generation who emerged with a higher sense of regeneration and symbiosis, and a spiritually activated practice for higher evolution.

CHAPTER 1

REWILDING DEFINED

Rewilding is an ancient concept being revived and reimagined in our modern context. The concept is sometimes polarizing, and the word is defined in various ways.

Purists speak of rewilding as the ultimate pursuit of living in full harmony with nature. They call us to reclaim our birthright as wild humans who depend on and interact with the natural environment to procure all resources symbiotically with the earth. It's a romantic vision of humanity and can be an admirable undertaking.

For others, rewilding means integrating the practices of hunting, foraging, and gathering into their lifestyle.

On the other extreme, some equate the idea of rewilding with bio-hacking, a popular movement relying on technology to aid the quest for immortality. This camp focuses on merging human biology with robotics and is on the hunt for the singularity—future superintelligent machines. This is definitely my least favorite interpretation of rewilding.

As with most things, my relationship with this concept is somewhere in the middle. For me, *rewilding* is returning to nature while consciously participating with our technologically driven world. I focus on fundamental nature-based principles that have allowed humans to evolve while adapting to highly unnatural environments.

All living things require specific and common elements to survive and thrive. Humans need sunlight, fresh air, pure water, nourishing food, movement, earthing, and community. Today, we can now make the case for having the best of both worlds. If we practice rewilding, viewing ourselves as an integral part of all living ecosystems on the planet, we will be heading in the right direction.

So as we adapt to a rapidly changing world, we reconnect to nature and integrate technological growth to achieve all that is necessary for humans to advance the species.

This is a huge challenge. In many ways these are opposite aims. Wildness is taboo. It invokes certain social aspects of culture, the concept of death, sexuality, egalitarianism, management of bodily urges and processes, and many more aspects of the animal part of our being. These cannot be overlooked. When we embrace these challenging parts of our nature, when we get curious and become aware of them, when we create habits to engage with them, we can transcend to higher levels of living.

When we suppress and alienate these "uncomfortable" characteristics of our human nature, we cannot evolve. In short, rewilding blends the best of nature-based foundations with the best of technology to form an elevated example of a well-rounded *Homo sapiens*.

Mindset, Context, and Self-Care for Life

The most important goal with this program is to apply it. If you want the advice in the following pages to be effective, you will have to integrate it via lifelong habits. If you do that, you will be embarking on the path of self-management and health improvement.

We are living in an age of information overload. We have all the data we need to accomplish anything we want, including attaining robust health. The downside is that we live in a state of chronic information excess that makes us feel overwhelmed and unable to chart the path forward. We are caught in a constant battle for our attention. Distractions. Bells. Whistles. Endless avenues to explore. The health field bombards us with claims about the next thing that will heal us. For example, there is a huge market right now for electronic wearables. These offer an endless supply of charts, measurements, and complex equations to describe our body's function in great detail.

The irony is that the constant monitoring of our body through these devices becomes disordered, making us reliant on this technology. People become dependent on a phone, watch, or other device to tell them what and how much to eat, when to exercise, when to go to the bathroom, and how many steps their bedtime routine should have in order to get the best sleep. After a while, people lose their sense of self, they become disconnected from the wisdom of the body. They find themselves more lost than when they began, so they give up.

Unfortunately, we've been conditioned to search for a quick fix or some magic pill. Most people have been convinced to trust superficial images and online anecdotes that, more often than not, distort the truth. We see this every day on social media, where thousands of influencers rely on filters, Photoshop, and unnatural posing to give the impression that a fairytale life is real. But it's not real.

It's time to get real. If we want to take back our health, reconnect with our bodies, and rewild our lives in this post-COVID world, we have to reject the idea of the magic pill and the quick fix. Tune in to your desire to succeed. Develop a growth mindset. Lean in to your innate adaptability. And commit yourself to lifelong learning.

Self-Care: Is It a Buzzword or a Legitimate Pursuit?

The messaging around achievement in our society has become wildly polarized. On the one end, we hear a lot about self-care. The loudest voices speak of self-care in terms of beauty and superficial appearance. On the opposite end of the spectrum, people preach extreme achievement: hustle, don't take a day off, push yourself to the limits. These are appropriate in certain contexts, of course, but taken as a model for life, these lead to dysfunctional patterns and chronic stress.

So, how can we take a more holistic approach to self-care? It is time to reclaim this word, to identify the ideals and practices we can look to in support of loving and compassionate care of the Self.

Today we are surrounded by unnatural elements. We have created environments that are challenging and unfit for the species. Our homes often have off-gassing persistent organic pollutants from furniture, carpets, fragrances from plug ins, etc. We consume our water from plastic bottles, increasing our exposure to endocrine disruptors. Chemicals and pollution abound. Artificial magnetic and electromagnetic fields increasingly affect our biology. Our food is often toxic and nutrient poor. The list goes on.

Self-care has to mean more than giving yourself a facial and going to yoga twice a week. Sustainable and effective self-care must take into account the requirements of our bodies in this altered environment.

Our goal is to organically and (over time) effortlessly create lifelong habits that will support a healthy and robust immunity for life.

Context Is Key

In my years in the wellness field, I have noticed a troubling trend. It's what Coach Scott Abel calls "the North American diet mentality." It's an unfortunate reality because, although diets today—with their extreme and polarizing concepts, fads, and empty promises—are very effective in selling books and products, they usually fail to move the masses toward health. Collectively, we have lost the value of common sense, which often happens when an idea or initiative is taken out of context. When considering a holistic and balanced approach to helping yourself and others, context is key.

We have to be aware that no one approach to eating is going to fit everybody. We have to factor in epigenetic history and lifestyle inputs. We also have to consider age, levels of activity, specific factors pertaining to where we live, how much we work, and the quality of our sleep. Therefore, it is imperative that we approach this program with context in mind.

I want to start by creating a strong foundation that applies to most people. This foundation is based on our evolution as hunter-gatherers who have emerged as a diverse species in the modern world still connected to the ecological cycle. Therefore, these pillars are centered around the elements of air, water, earth, fire, and ether.

Every species on the planet depends on these elements; humans are no exception. We were designed to breathe pure fresh **air** to improve oxygenation of the whole body. Clean **water** and clean, nutrient-dense food (**earth**) are essential for growth and regeneration. We rely on our sun (**fire**) for warmth, fuel, and light. The **ether** brings everything together and highlights our spiritual essence. By integrating these key elements, we learn to adjust, customize, and modify our needs and behaviors to match ever-changing circumstances. Context is key.

As you move through the following chapters, keep in mind the action steps below.

Action Steps

- Set up your mindset from the start. The advice in the following pages will require you to take action on the new principles you're learning. Don't let yourself get overwhelmed. Do your best at every step without expecting perfection. Aim to create lifelong habits over time.

- Get clear on what self-care means. Self-care goes beyond vanity and buzzwords. It is an aspect of your life that deserves awareness. Aim for restoration and recovery.

- Focus on context. Context and self-awareness are essential in discussing your health. Start by keeping a journal or taking notes about where you are in your health journey and where you want to go. Set realistic goals. Factor in your particular situation around work, family, and general lifestyle.

- Build strong foundations. This is critical for success. Master one new habit at a time. Explore one new concept at a time. This will allow you to apply what you're learning and avoid overwhelm.

CHAPTER 2

FOUNDATIONS

Survival of the fittest has been the dominant force throughout history, leading humans down a path of never-ending competition. It's the paradigm that has brought war, misunderstanding, and ever-present conflict.

We always seem to be fighting something. There was the war on drugs, then the war on terror, and now we are in the throes of the war against the virus. I believe that this concept has led us astray. Humans are not meant to merely survive. We have been designed through innovation and symbiotic relationships to cooperate in order to thrive in all environments. We are perhaps the most adaptable species on the earth. We owe this primarily to our fundamental interactions with the natural elements that fuel our bodies, minds, and spirits. Now more than ever, we must recapture our reliance on these foundations.

Sunlight and Natural Rhythms

*When the sun is shining I can do anything; no mountain
is too high, no trouble too difficult to overcome.*
–Wilma Rudolf, Olympic gold medalist and
fastest woman in the world, 1960

As the sun rises, so does all life on the planet. Today, however, many people fear the sun. Where did the fear of the sun come from? If we follow big business and massive, clever marketing campaigns, we can easily obtain clues. Did you know that the incidences of most health challenges were a lot less prevalent before we started putting unnatural chemicals and toxic substances on our skin? In 2019, *JAMA* published a preliminary study pointing to four sunscreen chemicals that were tested and found to enter the bloodstream, surpassing the levels FDA considered to be safe.[1]

Should we really be afraid of the sun, or is it just a convenient message encouraged by companies with a vested interest in perpetuating that fear?

The Body's Natural Clock

The sun powers every organism on earth and it is an essential figure in regulating our natural clock and daily rhythms. In simple terms, we rise with the sun and we set with the sun. Today we take this highly important detail for granted. Excess blue light from our devices, which we revere and depend on, has drastically upset our natural cycles. This has led to near epidemic levels of sleep imbalances. In turn, poor sleep health can negatively affect our mood, energy, hormonal function, blood sugar regulation, and even satiety—leading to weight gain.

The consequences and negative health implications deserve attention. We begin by addressing the retinal pathway of the eyes as it relates to light and dark cycles regulated by melatonin. Exposing our eyes to at least five minutes of morning sun daily will initiate the full cycle of melatonin that peaks in the evening. This in turn optimizes the natural hormone cycle.

"The circadian clock is the internal timing system that interacts with the timing of light and food to produce our daily rhythms. Our job is to maintain the clock so we can live with optimal health,"[2] explains Dr. Satchin Panda, author of *The Circadian Code.*

---

1 Murali K. Matta et al., "Effect of Sunscreen Application under Maximal Use Conditions on Plasma Concentration of Sunscreen Active Ingredients: A Randomized Clinical Trial," *JAMA* 321, no. 21 (2019), 2082–2091, doi:10.1001/jama .2019.5586.

2 Satchin Panda, PhD, *The Circadian Code: Lose Weight, Supercharge Your Energy, and Transform Your Health* (Emmaus: Rodale, 2018).

When you start the day off in order to calibrate hormones with the solar cycle, do not allow anything to block your eyes from sunlight. This includes sunglasses, prescription glasses, and contact lenses. Don't look directly at the sun, but stand in direct sunlight and gaze in the direction of the sun. A minimum of 5–15 minutes should be enough to receive the benefits.

This habit syncs your biological clock to that of the natural solar cycle. This in turn dictates a proper hormonal release throughout the day, ending with the critical release of melatonin at night.

Our bodies have multiple "clocks." Starting the day by syncing to the solar cycle allows all of them, not just the main one via the hypothalamus gland, to run in a harmonious and optimal way. There is a delicate cascade of timing to these clocks. The thyroid, for instance, manages metabolism; thus, proper signals from this highly important gland have to be in tune to set the timing sequence in motion. It's akin to a GPS being off by a millisecond. As this discrepancy increases, it builds and affects coordinates and direction, preventing the vehicle from arriving at its correct destination. In a similar way, our rhythms create a natural dopamine and serotonin ebb and flow that allows for consistent energy, appropriate biological processes, and stable moods.

After the morning cycle has been corrected, the next part of the equation is to get as much moderate sun exposure as possible throughout the day. All UVA, UVB, and UVC light works synergistically to optimize hormone function and natural vitamin (hormone) D production. In pre-modern times, aside from cultures living in predominantly cold climates, most humans did not rely on the use of excessive clothing. Our skin was naturally exposed to the full spectrum of light coming from our sun.

Misconceptions about Ultraviolet Light

There are three main frequencies of the UV spectrum that affect our biology via the eyes and skin: UVA, UVB, and UVC. All of these, contrary to popular belief, play an intricate and key role in the health of our biophoton capabilities, vitamin D absorption, cell function, and overall immunity.

Typically, we hear how UVB is dangerous and must be blocked. Most sunscreens are designed to block UVB rays in order to "protect" us from the harmful radiation. The reality is that our skin and biological systems are so sophisticated that they will naturally signal our body when it's had too much sun. Pigmentation and levels of melanin are evolutionary adaptations to help the skin shield against excessive rays, depending on longitude and proximity to the equator; this varies and creates an adequate mechanism of protection. Furthermore, we typically have an innate sense of our body's needs and capacity. We can feel that the body is getting burned if we expose ourselves for too long.

Skin pigmentation via melanin production has a self-regulating mechanism that not only protects our skin but also helps us adapt to environmental factors such as equatorial latitudes and higher sun exposure areas. In the past, as people settled and traveled further north and away from the sun, the skin became lighter with successive generations. In this way, these adaptations created a more effective mechanism for absorbing solar nutrients where levels of light are lower. So people with darker skin will typically be able to handle more sun while people with lighter skin may have decreased tolerance. All these factors, when given the right context, play a key role in getting nourished and balanced by the sun and trusting your body to regulate how much sunlight is best for you instead of covering your skin in sunscreen.

Bearing that in mind and considering the levels of individual pigmentation, we can use common sense and reconnect to the wisdom of our bodies in order to avoid these potentially harmful chemicals.

Blocking the body's self-regulating mechanism with chemical-based lotions prevents us from accessing this innate information. Furthermore, we have a good amount of evidence that UV light is a strong combatant against excessive viral load.

The use of sunscreen is a complex topic since we've been told it's safe. Sometimes we take issues like this at face value without doing a bit more research. My concern is that the reliance on sunscreen can lead to accumulation of some of the active ingredients. The *JAMA* study I mentioned earlier demonstrated the need for further testing on the cumulative effect of sunscreen use:

> In this preliminary study involving healthy volunteers, application of 4 commercially available sunscreens under maximal use conditions resulted in plasma concentrations that exceeded the threshold established by the FDA for potentially waiving some nonclinical toxicology studies for sunscreens.[3]

You might think, *Well, that sounds good, but what if I'm fair skinned and I want or have to be exposed to the sun for long periods of time?* Or you might wonder, *But what about my kids?* These are important and valid questions. Again, context is key. I naturally have darker, tan skin because I'm from the coast of Colombia near the equator. My four kids have a similar skin tone. Therefore, we can handle a bit more sun, whereas someone with fair skin will notice that their body is reacting to sun exposure more quickly.

Remember that context matters and every person should evaluate healthy sun exposure on a case-by-case basis. In general, though, I typically recommend the following best practices if you're going to be in direct sunlight for a long period, as you would at the beach or a pool.

---

3   Murali K. Matta et al., "Effect of Sunscreen Application under Maximal Use Conditions on Plasma Concentration of Sunscreen Active Ingredients: A Randomized Clinical Trial."

- Have cover available. Make sure you can access tents, canopies, or umbrellas so that you can control appropriate sun exposure.

- Bring suitable clothes. If you know you'll be outside well beyond your saturation point, or if you have a lighter skin tone and cannot tolerate long exposure, rely on clothing to cover exposed skin. This might be a breathable long-sleeve shirt, a swim coverup, or lightweight pants. Remember to bring a hat too.

- Slowly expand your tolerance. Over time you can build a solar "callus" by getting short bursts of sun exposure daily to increase melanin in the skin.

- Go organic. If you must use something on the skin for protection, go with organic, natural, and nontoxic sunscreen. Some people even use things like shea butter to ease the effects of longer time under the sun.

So, use common sense, check in with your body, and rely on appropriate cover when you need it. It's almost never a good idea to avoid the sun daily and expect that we can tan and toast ourselves on the beach over the weekend without skin damage. This is even more relevant when there is polyunsaturated fatty acids (PUFA) accumulation from most modern diets—more on this later.

Considering Blue Light Toxicity

Returning to the concept of energy, hormone function, and proper circadian rhythms, we need to consider the effects of excessive blue light exposure at night. Blue and green light are frequencies of the light spectrum that are most appropriate during the day—especially coming from the sun.

When the sun sets, blue light is no longer available naturally. Blue light exposure during the night from artificial sources such as tablets, smartphones, and TV screens creates a false impression of daylight. It fools our bodies into thinking that it still has time to be active and release adrenaline and cortisol. It also creates a challenging mismatch to our natural melatonin cycles. Moreover, it disrupts our natural rest cycle and interferes with proper and deep sleep. During the night is when most of our biological recovery occurs. Natural growth hormone, cellular, and tissue regeneration happen at this time as well.

Studies have illustrated the negative effects of blue light toxicity. One study published in Public Library of Science (PLoS) in 2011 showed that long periods of night shift work were associated with a modest increased risk in type 2 diabetes in women, which seems to be partially buffered through body weight.[4] This is similar to examples seen with night shift nurses working in hospitals, who typically show tendencies toward metabolic dysfunction, weight gain, blood sugar dysregulation, insomnia, and poor energy balance.

These unnatural environmental cues can weaken the immune system. Improper sleep and hormone dysfunction lead to inflammation, and chronic stress leads to massive magnesium deficiencies. Again, this creates enzyme function challenges that disrupt digestion, immunity, blood sugar control, and a host of other elements that downregulate the whole system.

What can you do about this?

1. Get morning sun.

As mentioned before, one of the best habits to create is to expose your eyes, unblocked, to morning sunlight in order to calibrate all biological clocks at the start of your day. Remember to shoot for at least 5–15 minutes and to also get as much on your skin as possible.

---

4   An Pan et al., "Rotating Night Shift Work and Risk of Type 2 Diabetes: Two Prospective Cohort Studies in Women," *PLOS Medicine*, December 6, 2011, https:// doi.org/10.1371/journal.pmed.1001141.

2. Get more sun when it matters most.

Depending on your skin tone, ethnicity, and where you live, try to find what your real solar time is and get moderate sun exposure between the hours of 11 a.m. and 12:30 p.m. Typically, this will be around 15 to 40 minutes, depending on the individual. A cool app you can use to get this information is called dminder.[5] But intuition and common sense are always there to guide you.

3. Block all blue light at night!

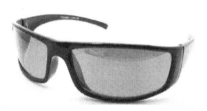

Humans evolved to rely on a natural source of light at night—fire. Avoid blue light at night and, if you need light, try red light. Studies are now showing that the infrared and red frequency of the light spectrum does not interfere with our natural cycles. Further, it is shown to have regenerative and beneficial effects for our overall health. Therefore, simulating amber candlelight at night can be healthy and fun.

Try wearing blue light blocking glasses at night. These amber or red lens glasses do a pretty good job of blocking almost 100% of the blue and green light coming from lightbulbs and our devices.

Also, downloading software like Iris[6] and f.lux[7] for laptops and computers is very helpful. This cool technology actually pairs our devices to sunset and automatically turns the blue light into a more reddish or amber color. Also, most smartphones and new tablets now come with blue light blocking options that can be found in the settings. These are free and easy ways to minimize blue light.

---

5   http://dminder.ontometrics.com

6   https://iristech.co

7   https://justgetflux.com

4. Shut everything down!

Ideally, we want to turn off all lights and/or use something like candlelight for lighting at night. The skin also has photo receptors that capture blue light and can contribute to blue light toxicity even while wearing the blue blocking glasses. Consider installing amber red bulbs at home and using those at night.

These things may not seem like a big deal. You might think that current lighting is just a part of our modern way of life, but remember that most of our technology has not been properly assessed for health outcomes. There are consequences to these changes; modeling our modern environment on a natural template is always best.

Takeaways

- Our hormones and circadian rhythms are vital for proper metabolism and overall immune function.
- It's extremely important to create habits that will return our hormones to a natural state related to the solar cycles.
- Get more sunshine in the morning and at midday.
- Block all artificial blue light at night.
- Refer to the numbered list right before these bullets to form lifelong habits.

CHAPTER 3

AIR AND BREATH MATTER

Most ancient and traditional systems of health value the integration of the five key elements of life. We will expand on water and earth (food) later. We covered the element of fire by highlighting the effects of the sun and circadian rhythms. This chapter highlights the importance of the air element. Proper blood flow and oxygenation are a critical part of regulating the immune system and supporting a long and healthy life.

Taking Control

The air we breathe has become toxic. Air quality is far from ideal: Exhaust from vehicles. Endocrine disruptors from artificial fragrances. Off-gassing from plastics, household products, and industrial processes. We have little control over these environmental toxins. When you add in the influence of mold, industrial chemicals, and paint fumes (the list goes on), you can see how we have managed to build a perfect storm of poor air quality.

Breathing high-quality oxygenated air is vital for cellular function, good metabolism, and a system of exchange in our body that gives us energy.

So what can we control? We have control over the quality of air inside our homes and offices. Consider the following actions you can take to create and maintain good air quality in your home or office environment.

Add Plants

The easiest and best place to start is to add plants in your home and office. These allies help clear out some of the debris and mitigate the organic pollutants mentioned above. Some of the most powerful plants that help clean up the air are snake plant, aloe vera, English ivy, flamingo lily, lady palm, Chinese evergreen, Kimberly Queen ferns, and bamboo palm.

Eliminate Toxins

Another factor that is simple, but often overlooked, is to take inventory of your home. Start to slowly eliminate anything that is not natural and creates toxic fumes and off-gassing. These can include but are not limited to fragrance plug ins, chemical-based cleaners and detergents, and other chemical-based airborne toxicants. Two good website that cover this in more detail with bullet points and videos are Wellness Mama[8] and Branch Basics.[9]

Add MOSO Bags

Another inexpensive and very helpful tool you can use in your home to cleanse toxic air is charcoal bags like MOSO bags. The charcoal in these bags is designed to absorb some of these compounds. Once a month, you discharge it under the sun.

Keep It Clean

Make sure your house is dust-free and kept clean. Your AC unit should be checked for proper flow, and a good filtration system should be in place.

---

8   https://wellnessmama.com/349305/home-microbiome/

9   https://branchbasics.com/home-cleanse/

Get a Filter

Finally, a good HEPA air filter system is an excellent investment for long-term care and improving overall circulation in the home. Even the more inexpensive units are effective. Just be sure they have HEPA, UV sanitizer, activated charcoal, and an ionizing feature. Some of my favorite brands are Air Oasis,[10] Guardian Technologies,[11] and TaoTronics.[12]

You and the people you love don't have to be passive about air quality. Use the advice above to take one small step at a time toward getting clean air quality. Your body will thank you and you'll be on your way to long-term health.

---

10   https://www.airoasis.com

11   https://amzn.to/2RtSfU6

12   https://amzn.to/32tJWhl

CHAPTER 4

PRISTINE WATER, HYDRATION, AND MINERALS

Water is the lifeblood of the planet and is essential to our body's functioning. Depending on a person's age and other factors like activity level and diet, we are designed to be 65–80% water. It is crucial to consume pristine and biologically appropriate water, as it directly interacts with our blood plasma, drives living ecosystems, and is the most natural.

Impure Drinking Water

In an ideal world, a natural source of water is wild, produced by nature, and created from deep underground aquifers untouched by pollution or human influence. It comes up through the earth in perfect form via true natural springs (sometimes called fossil water). Unfortunately, since the Industrial Revolution, the planet's hydrological cycle has been adversely modified. As a result of acid rain, agricultural runoff, fracking, glyphosate, leached plastics, and the heavy use of chemicals, these pristine springs no longer exist. As a result, most people end up consuming what we call hard water. *Hard water* is typically heavy in dissolved solids (inorganic and/or excess minerals) that can accumulate in our tissues. Our natural filtration system, the kidneys, can become overwhelmed and deposits of these dissolved solids accumulate.

Tap or municipal water has been improperly processed and presents many challenges. The Environmental Working Group, an activist group specializing in research and advocacy for clean water, writes,

"The inexcusable failure of the federal government's responsibility to protect public health means there are no legal limits for more than 160 unregulated contaminants in U.S. tap water."[13]

We have seen some improvements in water technology over the years, but most options still fail to achieve truly pristine and bioavailable water. We're ingesting substances every day that don't belong in our bodies and that cause us harm over time.

> EWG's Tap Water Database collects data from nearly 50,000 local utilities in 50 states – everything their required annual tests found in your community's drinking water. The disturbing truth shown by the data is that when most Americans drink a glass of tap water, they're also getting a dose of industrial or agricultural contaminants linked to cancer, harm to the brain and nervous system, changes in the growth and development of the fetus, fertility problems and/ or hormone disruption.[14]

Today's municipal water is lacking the intricate living elements and intelligence found in natural water. Most is improperly treated and infused with fluoride, chlorine, chloramine, heavy metals, etc. It has a molecular structure that lacks a proper hexagonal pattern and its molecules are too large. The water has sulfuric, nitric, and other acids that further degrade the pipes and your body and is not truly miscible with the blood. All these factors make it difficult for the body to achieve proper hydration, transport, and assimilation of nutrients through cellular membranes. It also makes it more challenging to flush or wash out toxins from the body.

Furthermore, most of these municipal water choices have a cationic or chaotic spin to them (down and out), which can create dysbiosis (improper bacterial balance), water retention, and overall biochemical

---

13   "The Dirty Secret of Government Drinking Water Standards," EWG, December 2019, https://www.ewg.org/tapwater/state-of-american-drinking-water.php.

14   "The Dirty Secret of Government Drinking Water Standards," EWG.

disruption. All water is best consumed totally free from all toxins, in an anionic pattern that's spinning up and in, and with proper mineralization (bicarbonates).

Glen Caulkins is one expert in this field I have been following for years. Glen has been working in the wellness field for over seventeen years and at age sixty-six he runs circles around most people half his age. His 180 IQ and masterful study of the human body; geological cycles of the planet; modalities such as chiropractic, spinal decompression, and clinical deep tissue massage; and the biosphere and the biogeochemical cycles have made him a pioneer and innovator in the development of water technology and overall health modalities.

Here's how Caulkins defines tap water: "acidic and chemically treated lifeless water that contains many contaminants including sulfuric, nitric, hydrofluorosilicic, haloacetic, hypochlorous, and hydrochloric acids; fluoride, heavy metals, chlorine/chloramine, disinfectant byproducts, pharmaceuticals, etc."[15]

Glen Caulkins's research is invaluable for those who want to know what they're putting in their bodies. He has managed to create a true solution for our times. This is one of the reasons why, after all my years in the wellness field, I still use and recommend his system, which we'll discuss in the next section, as the best water option above all others.

Finding Your Clean Water Source

Make finding a clear water source a priority right now. We are meant to be 65–80% saline-solution beings, so it is critical that we consider the best strategy for getting clean water. This applies not only to drinking, but also to food preparation, cooking, and bathing. Think about it this way: if you take care of your water strategy, you're taking care of at least 65% of your overall health equation.

---

15   "Your Current Drinking Water Options Explained," Live Pristine, accessed November 20, 2020, https://livepristine.com/blogs/news-views/your-current-drin king-water-options-explained.

Of course, I always encourage you to do your own research and learn about this topic for yourself. But I'm here to share with you what I know. Through many years of researching how to get clean water, I have tried pretty much all water options available. Although I've come across some good solutions, the revival system recommended here is by far the best and most complete solution. It's a ten-stage process that offers pristine, highly structured, oxygenated, sustainable water rich in magnesium bicarbonate and hydrogen from the convenience of your home.

This technology is called PristineHydro.[16] The system goes beyond reverse osmosis (RO), distillation, and water ionizing, and is superior to plastic/stale/overly priced spring and other bottled waters. It overcomes every obstacle in order to create the highest-quality water for nourishing your body.

Daily Water Intake

Should we drink the recommended eight glasses of water a day? The short answer is … it depends. Pay attention to your water needs. In addition to the more common chronic problem of dehydration—not drinking enough water—there is such a thing as drinking too much water. Excessive fluid consumption—known as hypernatremia—can create a loss of sodium inside the cell. This creates an electrolyte imbalance; it can lead to cramping and even to such a high level of mineral deficiency that it can affect proper overall function of the body. Again, balance is key and no one formula fits all. Things to consider: height, weight, activity levels, how much other fluids you are taking, electrolyte balance, etc. Are you eating enough salt? How much do you sweat? Are there enough minerals coming in through nutrition?

---

16   https://pristinehydro.com

A Final Piece of Advice on Water

Stop drinking from plastic bottles right now. Get with the glass! This is critically important because plastic has bisphenols (BPA) that act as endocrine disruptors. While you may know about the dangers of BPA, you may not be familiar with the effects of photodegradation. Bottled water that is stored at warm temperatures and is exposed to direct sunlight creates a form of oxidation as the polymers and other plastics degrade—much like paintings and other artifacts are damaged when exposed to excessive light and air. In other words, it breaks down the plastic bonds, and the estrogen-like materials leach into the water, creating a type of hormone disruptive "tea."

Get the Full Story on Salt

For many people, the subject of salt can be quite confusing and even controversial. It's understandable, considering that the mainstream medical community often blames salt for things like high blood pressure. When we consider highly processed and prepackaged foods with extreme levels of sodium, we can see the possibility of ingesting unnatural levels of sodium over time.

Ironically, however, proper levels of sodium and potassium and an overall balance of minerals in the body are exactly what the body needs to regulate blood pressure, proper circulation, and general mitochondrial function. Salt is also necessary for digestion and the proper production of hydrochloric acid. HCL is extremely important for the breakdown of nutrients in the body, especially protein, and it's one of the body's first lines of defense against bacteria, viruses, and other unwanted pathogens.

Pure Sea Salt

In the absence of trace minerals, plain (stripped) sodium chloride can present challenges. Pure sea salt has trace elements that allow for the bicarbonate cycle (in water) to generate energy and a proper electrical circuit. This is one of the main reasons salt is so vital. In my years in the wellness field, the people I have noticed to display signs of imbalance are those who overly restrict salt. They tend to have a dry complexion, poor energy, erratic mood due to improper brain function, and general body weakness.

So, it's good to eat salt in moderate amounts. I recommend choosing pure white sea salt without anything added.

Himalayan or pink salt is very popular. It is often touted as a miracle salt offering trace elements. The challenge with this type of salt is that its red color comes from excess iron, which can create a rusting effect. Over time, this will accumulate in the body and disrupt cell function. Also, it's a rock salt, which can lead to rock formations (crystals) inside the body as well.

Gray salts tend to have excess tin; these also tend to accumulate. I used the grey Celtic sea salt for years but switched to the more purified type when I discovered I had tin accumulation. Unfortunately, until our oceans are allowed to fully regenerate, these "natural salts" should be used sporadically.

There are many exotic and "therapeutic" salts on the market. Although these could be fun and have a cool culinary and tonic effect, I advise against using them as a staple salt. Again, pure white sea salt is my choice for the time being.

As you can see, water, salt, and mineral balance is an extremely important part of the whole health equation. Yet, it's an aspect that is overlooked. Being water-based creatures, our collagen integrity, immune function (via cytoplasm, the gel-like matrix inside and outside the cells), and mitochondria (the electrical component) are all mediated by water.

Nourishment through food, which is the next major piece of the puzzle, is dependent in many ways on the quality and integrity of water.

CHAPTER 5

FOOD FOUNDATION

What is nourishment?

nour·ish·ment
/ˈnəriSHmənt/

Noun

1. *The food or other substances necessary for growth, health, and good condition.*

Synonyms
nutrition – food – nutriment – aliment – sustenance[17]

If we were to go by these basic definitions, then our eating paradigm should be quite simple. And, in a way, it is. The bare bones answer is that we should eat whatever we recognize as "real food," meaning that it comes from nature. Unfortunately, modern life has made our food web reliant on a profit-driven industry that produces unnatural, highly processed food. This environment requires us to develop a more complex strategy for obtaining the nourishment we need.

Real Food: What's In and What's Out?

Our current brain size, species behavior, and physiological progression are the product of our evolution; we are a hunter-gatherer society. We hunt animal protein of different sorts (wild game, beef, poultry, fish and seafood). What do we gather? Fruits, vegetables, eggs, root vegetables and tubers, and small amounts of nuts and seeds.

---

17 *Oxford University Press*, Lexico.com, accessed November 23, 2020, s.v. "nourishment," https://www.lexico.com/en/definition/nourishment.

You may be thinking, *Oh no, not another primal/paleo diet.* Don't worry, this isn't that. The foods mentioned above are meant only as a strong foundation—a starting point that provides a solid basis of nourishing, nutrient-dense, and calorie-appropriate foods. These foods should be the staples of our diet. Today we have the luxury of adding more variety by including high-quality full-fat dairy, legumes, and wild grasses (grains).

Apart from these, some "foods" should be considered rare options while others should be avoided altogether. These come mostly from laboratory settings where humans, not nature, have attempted to improve the food supply. So far, we have fallen short of the mark. Highly processed foods are the major culprits behind many of our primary health challenges today. We'll discuss this in more detail toward the end of the chapter.

What does it mean to eat real food? It means prioritizing foods that you recognize as being harvested in their whole state from the earth. We're talking about food sources that were once living. The main kingdoms of food you want to include are plants, animals, fungi (mushrooms), and bacteria (cultured foods). For simplicity's sake I'm including algae (seaweed) as part of the plant kingdom even though these are a kingdom of their own. Remember, if you don't recognize the food as naturally occurring or you can't pronounce the items in the ingredient list, think twice before consuming it!

The Plant Kingdom

Most people likely get the bulk of their calories from the plant kingdom. This kingdom comprises vegetables, fruits, roots and tubers, nuts, seeds, legumes, whole grains, herbs, spices, and sea vegetables. This presents us with endless possibilities and diverse choices and adds a great deal of color, nutrition, and creativity to our meals.

The Animal Kingdom

This kingdom comprises wild game, grass-fed free-ranging ruminants, pork, fowl, fish and seafood, eggs, dairy products, and even insects. This is perhaps the kingdom of food that causes the most controversy. Opposing camps have an almost religious fervor for their respective food philosophies, making differences of opinion wildly polarized. For example, vegans—who abstain from consuming all animal foods—typically have major disagreements with carnivores, who prioritize eating animal foods. Both camps tend to be extreme and vocal about their diet's superiority, becoming locked in a battle of right and wrong. This arises from a major misunderstanding and disconnection from our natural ecosystems.

The question of animal rights and ethical treatment of animals is highly charged, which is understandable given our dysfunctional approach to animal husbandry. The factory farm infrastructure is infamous for its unethical treatment of animals and unsustainable practices. This has given rise to marketing campaigns calling for consumers to stop eating meat.

I don't wish to take sides in this particular debate. I will, however, say that nature works in a sophisticated death-and-life cycle. There is no way around it. One creature or plant has to die so that another can live. This is what makes humans an active participant of the ecology. Our choices matter. When we view our place on the planet as one within the living ecosystems, we realize that we are indeed part of nature. As a species we have a very long track record of fitting successfully within this equation. Only in recent history (because of the rise of irresponsible industrial processes) has our departure from this symbiotic relationship become a valid and necessary consideration.

The Fungi Kingdom

This kingdom comprises all types of edible mushrooms—excluding those that have been recognized as poisonous, highly toxic, or exhibiting hallucinogenic properties. Aside from these, we are left with a bounty of edible and medicinal mushrooms that offer great health benefits. A few popular examples of edible mushrooms are portobello, button, king oyster, white, and shiitake. Some of the more popular medicinal mushrooms are reishi, chaga, cordyceps, maitake, agaricus, and lion's mane. The medicinal mushrooms are important to the discussion of COVID; they are immune modulators with the ability to help naturally regulate the immune system.

The Bacteria Kingdom

This group offers us a unique tapestry of nutrients that are all too often ignored. Although the word "bacteria" carries a negative connotation in the Western world, it is a highly important food group that must be included in our diet. Incorporating the right cultures into our food can create a highly functioning inner ecosystem that is vital for achieving optimal health. We actually house more bacteria in our bodies than human cells. This is not a category to be underestimated. If you aren't in the habit of thinking of bacteria as food, think sauerkraut, kimchi, lacto-fermented dairy products, and coconut ferments. Our most popular condiments today such as ketchup, salsa, and mustard were originally used as cultured condiments. Further, in traditional cultures, these were fermented to aid in digestion.

I'd like you to consider that just because we now have all these choices available doesn't mean that we have to incorporate them into our diet. After all, nutrition is not the only reason we eat (right, foodies?). Moreover, due to individual situations, metabolic states, geographic location, and epigenetics, we all have different needs. A singular method is not meant to work for everyone.

Context is king!

In my specific case, for example, dairy products—apart from ghee, grass-fed low-temperature whey protein, farm fresh cottage cheese, and yogurt—typically don't provide me with optimal results. I also choose to abstain from pork. We are all different. We have to understand this fundamental truth if we are to shift to a healing paradigm.

Considering Calorie Intake

How much we should eat is another controversial issue in our society. Some people glorify the idea of eating light. Others demonize a sparse diet. The reality is that calories do matter to some extent. There are health authors, teachers, and presenters who have made careers from their claims that calories don't matter as long as you _____ (fill in the blank). Don't buy into the hype.

Again, context is king!

How active are you? Are you sitting most of the day? Are you an avid CrossFitter? Do you tend to overtrain? Do you have a history of chronic dieting? How is your metabolism? What does your relationship with food look like? What is your usual stress level? These are all important questions that will impact the amount of energy (calories) you need to consume per day. Just remember, your lifestyle should and probably already does dictate a lot of your food choices.

Of course there are other considerations that are part of the equation when constructing your diet: movement, proper hydration, stress management, and holistic lifestyle. You have all the information you could ever need on these topics at your fingertips. While that is a gift, it can also feel like a curse. Don't let the sheer volume of information overwhelm you. Take one piece of the puzzle at a time and play with all these wonderful concepts. Little by little, as you construct the puzzle of your overall health and well-being, the small daily changes you make will pave the way to vital health. It will no longer seem like a difficult goal or a fruitless endeavor.

I hope this short guide brings value and perspective to your life. At the very least, I hope it moves you closer to achieving a sense of balance and general well-being. Every one of us deserves to be well.

Enjoy your life, be happy, and eat well!

Check out the appendixes for guidance about how to clean your fridge and pantry and how to meal plan and create a recipe rotation.

CHAPTER 6

TOXICANTS OF THE MODERN AGE AND HOW TO AVOID THEM

The aspect of our society that has changed most dramatically is our environment. In the previous chapters, we discussed the ways humans have departed from the natural elements: We live primarily indoors, under artificial light, and without enough natural sunlight. We are not drinking pristine water. The food we eat and the air we breathe are less than ideal. Let's face it, we live in a massively toxic world. This environmental shift to a chemically based society is perhaps the biggest factor that has affected our biology. And, yes, it has potentially altered our interaction with the various strains of coronaviruses.

Our crops are laced with harmful chemicals, pesticides, herbicides, fungicides, Roundup (glyphosate+), and more. We are exposed to industry byproducts, plastics xenoestrogens, microplastics, pollutants from vehicle exhaust, and mercury in the ocean. The list goes on.

In agriculture the exclusive use of NPK (nitrogen, phosphorus, potassium) chemical fertilizers has disrupted the nitrogen cycle and the soil microbiome. This, in turn, has led to nutrient deficiencies (especially magnesium) and accumulation of calcium and acids.

Highly toxic elements like aluminum, cadmium, mercury, arsenic, lead, and other persistent organic pollutants have shown up in testing and actual cases of patients with Alzheimer's, cancer, diabetes, and cardiovascular challenges.

Specific to COVID, we have to factor in the effects of cyanide and glyphosate, as these two chemicals create a situation where the body becomes hypoxic, a low-blood-oxygen state due to poisoning. This, in turn, causes lung tissue to fill up with fluid. In the case of COVID, this means we have to consider a possibility that doesn't fit the narrative that this is an infection-based illness. For decades our ecosystems have been blanketed with glyphosate, a harmful pesticide that shows high probabilities of toxic accumulation.[18] When considering that the highest numbers of initial cases were discovered in high-pollution cities like NYC, northern Italy, Wuhan, and Ecuador, this explanation at the very least deserves a much closer look. For more resources on the toxicity of glyphosate in humans, see the References section at the end of the book. For a more in-depth discussion of the link between environmental toxicity and COVID-19, see Appendix D.

There are many ways this toxic accumulation disrupts our physiology. Dr. Joseph Pizzorno, author of *The Toxin Solution*, explains:

> When a chemical toxin enters your body, it actually alters the speed at which many key functions take place. This alteration can decrease the activity of the enzymes that are required for every bodily function. For example, toxins may:
>
> - Increase or decrease heart rate.
>
> - Interrupt neuron connections necessary for the brain to function.
>
> - Decrease the production of thyroid hormones that regulate how fast enzymes work.
>
> - Block insulin receptor sites on cells so sugar can't get in to produce energy.[19]

Although the body was originally designed and equipped to confront pollutants and toxins, our modern industrial landscape has

---

18 Stephanie Seneff et al., "Can glyphosate's disruption of the gut microbiome and induction of sulfate deficiency explain the epidemic in gout and associated diseases in the industrialized world?" *JBPC* 17 (2017).

19 Joseph Pizzorno, *The Toxin Solution* (New York: HarperCollins, 2017).

overloaded the body's ability to handle the load. We are now at a point where we must actively address this issue.

Consider the following solutions:

- Become aware of the presence of toxic overload and acknowledge it is of vital concern to address it.

- Shop local and organic as much as possible. Learn about and support the growing movement toward regenerative agriculture.

- Avoid gluten, found in grains like wheat, barley, spelt, kamut, triticale, and rye. The protein itself is inflammatory, and crops are subject to the spraying of massive amounts of glyphosate and Roundup. This seems to be the major culprit for the high incidence of gut perforation that is leading many into irritable bowel and autoimmune challenges.

- Avoid conventional dairy products from factory farms, which expose animals to excessive amounts of chemicals, antibiotics, and other unnatural ingredients that get transferred to the food they produce. The body's reaction to dairy varies from person to person and is influenced by epigenetics. If you consume dairy, prioritize healthy grass-fed dairy products; these have enzyme cofactors intact that can be potentially nutritious, especially in their raw form.

- Avoid farmed fish at all costs. The animals are confined, and their feed is highly contaminated, which is transferred into the animals' tissues. This is yet another source of the persistent organic pollutants we've talked about.

- Reduce your toxic load at home. I recommend you do a thorough inventory for mold and off-gassing elements from paint, carpets, modern furniture, etc. Invest in air-purifying plants and a good air filter.

- Reduce your use of personal care products like deodorant,

perfumes, and makeup that have aluminum and lead, or switch to nontoxic products.

- Purchase products stored in glass, stainless steel, or other materials that don't have toxic elements.

- Cook with stainless steel or ceramic, and avoid aluminum and nonstick cookware.

- Avoid plastics as much as possible, as they are major endocrine hormone disruptors.

- Learn more about safe, gentle, and natural detox strategies like infrared sauna and red light therapy.

Our environment and lifestyles have become disconnected from the natural world. The extreme use of artificial and highly toxic chemicals in our water, food, homes and offices, clothing, and almost all industrial-based businesses has created an environment requiring us to detox to maintain optimal health. We must learn new strategies and develop innovative ways to counter these assaults on our biological processes.

CHAPTER 7

MOVEMENT AND BODYWORK

Bodywork is one of the most powerful lifestyle practices that I've added into my routines and recommend to my clients. Apart from drinking clean water and getting optimal levels of magnesium, nothing can dissolve excess calcium deposits, fibrosis, and scar tissue better than bodywork. Waking up to the unnatural environment you're living in and addressing the effects to your body is a game-changing approach to health, wellness, and longevity.

Most people have no idea that their ill health is rooted in the negative effects of calcium deposits, fibrosis, and scar tissue accumulation. It's a massive oversight. Calcium deposits occur due to many factors. A big one is excess calcium that ends up in soft tissue instead of bone. This leads to muscular and overall body pain. It's like having little bits of coral in your tissues—it hurts when you put pressure on them. An extreme example of this is someone who suffers from arthritis. The deposits have become so excessive that the person loses movement and the joints fuse; they becomes stiff, almost rock like. Mineral imbalances and deficiencies, toxic accumulation, and advanced fibrosis also cause calcification. The good news is that calcium deposits are reversible.

Fibrosis is an inflammatory process that creates adhesions, fibroids, and hardened scar tissue. It creates a web-like effect in collagen (protein crosslinking) and leads to immobility and shortening of muscle and fascia. This creates a network of dysfunctional chains in the body, limits range of motion, and leads to excess accumulation of metabolic byproducts and calcium. The combination of bodywork with proper mineral balance, hydration, magnesium, and a few innovative ideas (which I'll introduce later) can equip the body to combat high toxic loads and strengthen the immune system.

Bodywork Defined

What is bodywork? Most people know about massage therapy, the most popular versions being Swedish, deep tissue, sports, shiatsu, reflexology, aromatherapy, and Thai massage. Although these are all excellent—especially for relaxation, lymphatic movement, and improving the nervous system—they're not at the same level of therapeutic bodywork I'm recommending in the context of this book.

As the word implies, bodywork in the context of deep rejuvenation is exactly that: work. It feels most like work for the patient in the beginning stages. The practice targets trigger points and aims to achieve myofascial release. Trigger points are akin to micro knots that form in the body. These often come about through injury or trauma, repetitive movements, chronic tightness, and improper warmup and form during training. Myofascial release is a method of reforming the collagen in the body through pinning muscle, shearing, mashing, and/or slow holds that lead to an almost melting effect. It's subtle but quite powerful.

It is very difficult to achieve healing in the tissues without undertaking the actual manual and physical practices that lead to dissolving calcium crystals, eliminating fibrosis, and unwinding tight or bound up fascia. For those living a predominantly sedentary life, muscles and connective tissues become shortened, constricted, less supple, and limited in range of motion. This eventually leads to dehydration, metabolic dysfunction, and chronic aches and pains, which contribute to lowered immunity.

Fascia Defined

What is fascia?

Fascia, in simple terms, is a complex matrix of collagen and interstitial fluid that acts as a webbing that surrounds all muscle, organs, and other tissues of the body. Fascia is three-dimensional and acts as a tensegrity structural system. This highly sophisticated system joins many components of the body that are under stress and tension while being perfectly arranged to hold and move us through space. Due to nutritional deficiencies, dehydration, deposits of inorganic minerals, and lack of natural movement, fascia can become stiff. It's like a sponge that doesn't get emptied out, or a shirt that is bunched up so that it restricts full range of motion. Fascia can also become limited in its ability to transport fluids and naturally detoxify the body. This affects proper immunity.

Tom Myers, author of *Anatomy Trains*, writes:

Fascia is the biological fabric that holds us together, the connective tissue network. You are about 70 trillion cells—neurons, muscle cells, epithelia—all humming in relative harmony; fascia is the 3D spider web of fibrous, gluey, and fascial wet proteins that binds them together in their proper placement. Our biomechanical regulatory system is highly complex and under-studied—though new research is filling in the gap. Understanding fascia is essential to the dance between stability and movement—crucial in high performance, central in recovery from injury and disability, and ever-present in our daily life from our embryological beginnings to the last breath we take.[20]

Cultivating a consistent bodywork practice and seeing a well-trained professional for regular sessions is an incredible strategy for optimal

---

20 Thomas W. Myers, *Anatomy Trains: Myofascial Meridians for Manual and Movement Therapists* (London: Churchill Livingstone, 2014).

health. Visit the Rewilding COVID[21] online interactive platform to watch videos about the best tools and routines for self-work in a range of price points. We also have videos available for partner work using what is called the GC (Glen Caulkins) Method. GC Method is one of my favorites because it empowers couples or friends to apply the bodywork on each other using a walker (to hold their own weight) to manipulate the tissues with the feet. This resource will be updated over time to include a list of practitioners that use these and similar methods.

I'm passionate about bodywork because of its effectiveness in healing dysfunction, eliminating pain, and optimizing health. Patients suffering back, neck, and knee pain will reap amazing benefits from bodywork. Athletes can benefit from these modalities to correct over-training and injuries. And sedentary people often present with imbalances in shortened hip flexors and bad posture, which can be improved with the use of bodywork.

Train Hard—Recover Harder!

The fitness industry has grown at an incredible rate in recent years. The big gyms, fitness chains, and extreme training concepts have benefitted most from this trend. Unfortunately, the average consumer has not reaped the rewards. We are not much closer to honing our bodies into truly "great shape."

Along with the industry's growth, messages abound: no days off, hustle hard, never give up, push through the pain. Social media platforms like Instagram present a false sense of beauty. My wish is to see more messages of self-empowerment, nuance and context, and balance.

As an example from my life, I'm a father of four and my youngest daughter is two. She sometimes has leg pains at night and may wake up crying two to three times per night. You won't be surprised to learn

---

21   Rewildingcovid.com

that my sleep patterns aren't ideal, and I wake up feeling tired. Instead of pushing myself to do the scheduled workout or movement session, I'll often opt for a recovery activity that doesn't build upon the stress of my specific situation. This might mean taking a long walk, choosing a self-bodywork routine, or even just resting more throughout the day. Furthermore, situations like these can sometimes lead to a bit of weight gain because of sleep interruption and the added stress. I choose to understand that this is a cycle in my life that will evolve; I try not to be too hard on myself and make matters worse.

This is why context is valuable. Self-love and personal awareness are the best guides to making choices about optimal health one day at a time. Toxic messages about beauty abound. The truth is that becoming aware, reconnecting to the wisdom of your body, and loving yourself makes you beautiful no matter your shape or size. As a society, we need to bring more awareness to the distortion of beauty via the reliance on technology, false ideals, and distorted images.

Our modern world fuels and sometimes even glorifies chronic and excessive stress. But stress has been linked to exhaustion, hormonal dysfunction, and almost all instances of ill health. In the context of exercise, counter to popular belief, more is not always better. Of course, we are designed to move and to use our bodies for many activities. However, our modern values of fitness have taken training and exercise out of context. Some people are overtraining when they should be resting. Most people lead a sedentary life during the week and then overextend themselves on the weekend. This perpetuates the cycle of stress and injury; it's an unsustainable lifestyle.

In order to cultivate a balanced approach to exercise, we have to understand the value of cycles. Our bodies operate on anabolic and catabolic processes. These cycles are used by the body to build up and break down in order to rebuild, grow, and become better. Here is where proper recovery via self-bodywork, stress management, rest, and good sleep become relevant. Meditation, tai chi, infrared sauna, float tanks, and other forms of "working in" are valuable too. And again, being mindful of cycles of more-vigorous versus less-intense forms of exercise is very important. Walking for medium to long distances is a tried and true but underrated form of movement that offers incredible benefits. For one, it's a low impact way of moving lymph throughout the body, which improves the immune system. In 2017 the *American Journal of Preventive Medicine* concluded that "Walking is simple, free, and does not require any training, and thus is an ideal activity for most Americans, especially as they age."[22]

Finally, new approaches to natural movements based on evolutionary principles are emerging. These are demonstrating that gait cycle, proper posture, and certain codes or patterns of movement present us with the proper antidote to the current mobility challenges we face today. Some of the concepts and systems leading the way to true innovation in fitness are Functional Patterns[23] and MovNat.[24]

Functional Patterns is a system of movement and training created by Naudi Aguilar based on the premise that humans were designed to walk, run, and throw. This innovative approach seeks to relieve dysfunctionality in humans by bringing them back to proper function in a methodical, challenging, and fun way. MovNat stands for natural movement and was created by Erwan Le Corre. He also created a system based on natural human movements like walking, crawling, climbing, running, and even some elements of parkour.

---

22   Alpa V. Patel, PhD et al., "Walking in Relation to Mortality in a Large Prospective Cohort of Older U.S. Adults," *AJPM* 54, no. 1 (January 2018), 10–19.

23   https://www.functionalpatterns.com

24   https://www.movnat.com

Tools

The following is a basic list of tools that I recommend for self-bodywork. These will support your efforts to maintain fascia, muscles, and overall body health.

- Lacrosse ball[25]
- Accumobility balls[26]
- Foam roller or PVC Pipe[27]
- Thera cane[28]
- Softball and baseball[29]
- Walker (for GC Method and partner myofascial release)[30]
- Hypervolt, Tim Tam, and other similar massage "guns"[31]

---

25 https://amzn.to/2Imi6wz

26 www.acumobility.com/?ref=61

27 https://amzn.to/3u02DFs

28 https://amzn.to/3eV4Smj

29 https://amzn.to/3lrj2xR

30 https://amzn.to/35mS1WK

31 https://amzn.to/2Np3yya

CHAPTER 8

GROUNDING AND THE
ELECTRICITY OF THE BODY

What are electromagnetic frequencies or fields (EMFs), and why are they important? Our bodies have an electromagnetic component that interacts with magnetic and electrical fields. Think about a patient getting an EKG in the hospital to read the electrical signals coming from their heart—that's a perfect example of how one device is interacting with the human electromagnetic component. Fields are created from electrical appliances, cell phones and cell towers, Wi-Fi, and even the natural magnetic field of the earth.

When our bodies interact with these external EMFs, our health is affected. This is yet another example of how humans are interacting with non-natural elements in their environment, becoming disconnected from the natural world. Effects of non-native or artificial EMFs on the body are similar to the effects of the sea of chemicals we've been exposed to since the Industrial Revolution. Even though we can't see these fields, they affect our biology. We can measure these electronic and magnetic fields to determine whether they are safe or potentially harmful.

Whether we like it or not, we all have to face the reality that we live in this sea of unnatural invisible frequencies that affect our biology. We're like fish swimming in polluted waters. Although we enjoy many benefits brought forth by our ever-advancing technologies, the consequences to human health have not been properly addressed. Let's face it, big tech and telecommunication companies are not going to risk their bottom line for people's health. So it is up to us to take charge; we have to take responsibility to safeguard our health. EMF and health expert Martin Pall, PhD, explains that EMFs "actually greatly increase the influx of calcium ions through these voltage-gated calcium channels.... Most, if not all, biological effects are produced by excessive intracellular calcium..."[32]

As Pall points out, calcification in the interior of the cell creates an effect similar to a traffic jam where everything becomes halted and function is impaired. In this way, EMFs affect mitochondria, cell function, and ratios of calcium in our bodies; it is a key component of our electrical matrix. The higher ratios of calcium in the cell destabilize its ability to keep its integrity. This excess calcium can also lead to vulnerability to infections or toxic accumulation of exosomes (virus) produced as a byproduct of the deficient and weakened cell.

Finding a Solution

There are many ways we can adapt to, mitigate, and at times even overturn the effects of EMFs. As always, begin by becoming aware that EMFs affect your health. From a place of awareness, you can engage in conversation with partners, friends, families, and community to create solidarity and work toward solutions. Don't allow yourself to become overwhelmed with the current state of exposure. Begin noticing and recording symptoms of EMF exposure. Some of the common symptoms are chronic fatigue, poor sleep/insomnia, memory loss, headaches, brain fog, anxiety, depression, heart palpitations, ongoing dizziness, and visual disruption due to light sensitivity.

Consider the following actions you can take to mitigate your exposure to EMFs:

1. Understand that distance is your friend. The farther you are from your phone, laptop, and other devices, the less direct exposure

---

32 Martin Pall, PhD, 5G Summit interview, June 17, 2020, https://www.youtube.com/watch?v=TtC6oHWjg7g.

you have against your body. This has an exponential effect, so the farther you can be without disrupting your effective use, the better. When taking a call, it's best to use a headset with an air tube or a regular headset—avoid using Bluetooth. Keep your phone away from your head at all times. This is especially important for children, as they're not fully developed (especially the brain). In an ideal world, children under the age of fifteen should have limited to no exposure to any of these devices. However, the reality is that technology has infiltrated our family lives. Those who allow their children access to devices can monitor use and ensure children only watch downloaded material on airplane mode.

2. Build habits to lessen exposure. The most important factor here is to shut off your Wi-Fi at night. You can develop the habit of turning it off before bed every night or set up an automatic timer that does it for you. You don't need the router on while you sleep.

3. Turn devices on airplane mode: while on your body, when not in use, and overnight. I also highly recommend that your phone be left out of the bedroom. If you use it as an alarm clock, I would still leave it outside and most definitely put it on airplane mode. With your phone, aside from the EMF factor, you also want to set up a shortcut[33] to manually put the phone on the red light screen before bed. If you absolutely do need the phone as an alarm and you keep it in your bedroom, then having the screen on red will ensure that blue light doesn't hit your eyes at the wrong times and disrupt your circadian rhythms.

4. Use mitigation technology and practices around your home and office. These include installing Stetzer filters and kill switches,

---

33 https://www.instagram.com/p/B2MfS5AokLl/?igshid=14xzzz8rwqv0g

or finding the breakers for your bedroom and getting the house or office hardwired ethernet.

5. Bonus step: Identify how many cell towers or 5G towers are close to your home or office and how far away they are. This is extremely important. Unfortunately, if you are sensitive to the EMFs created by these towers and they're too close, I recommend moving to another home or office as soon as circumstances allow.

6. Bonus step: This step is based on the concept of the scalar energetic effects of EMFs. Scalar energy is characterized by its subtle and coherent wave patterns, which mimic natural fields. Using technology like a Blushield Cube that interrupts the software or information packets of non-native frequencies has been shown to be beneficial in offsetting the negative impact of EMFs. Blushield[34] is a company that has figured out a way to go beyond simple EMF remediation. In other words, their technology creates algorithms and resonant frequencies that overpower the artificial and potentially harmful waves we are exposed to from cell phones, Wi-Fi, etc. This can become a bit complicated and it is a difficult sell because of lack of research. However, many anecdotal accounts and measured biological results have demonstrated some positive effects, so if you can afford the investment, this option is worth exploring.

For a much more developed strategy to optimize your home and or office, it's best to measure the frequencies being emitted. Here are a few meter suggestions and videos on how to do it yourself:

- ENV RD-10 3-Mode Compact EMF Meter[35]
- Shielded Healing ESI 24 Meter[36]

---

34 https://www.blushield-us.com/?ref=84

35 https://amzn.to/3kGlsqp

36 https://shieldedhealing.com/products/esi-24-emf-meter

- Luke Storey's EMF Home Safety Master Class[37]

It would be ideal to hire an EMF expert or building biologist. Shielded Healing is an EMF mitigation and measuring site developed by Brian Hoyer. Brian is one of the top experts on measuring EMFs in the home and creating strategies to improve the electronic environment at home and in the office. He is my top recommendation for this service.

Another great resource is the Building Biology Institute, which aims to create healthy homes by using principles of nature. Their designs take into account indoor air, tap water pollutants, mold, and hazards from electromagnetic radiation. They also have a list on their site of highly trained professionals[38] who can make thorough assessments of your home and office.

Grounding with Nature

The subject of grounding or earthing is sometimes critiqued as being unscientific. But our species evolved walking on the earth in our bare feet, grounded to the earth's native electromagnetic frequency. By being barefoot on the surfaces of the earth (soil and water are conductive materials), we actually receive an influx of what's called spare electrons that actively help heal inflammation and improve immunity.

Regardless of what critics say, a growing body of research supports this phenomenon, showing that grounding helps improve the biological processes in our body.[39,40] It does this primarily by creating a natural anti-inflammatory reaction. The natural current of the earth offsets an

---

37   https://online.lukestorey.com/emf-class/

38   https://buildingbiologyinstitute.org/find-an-expert/

39   James L Orschman, Gaetan Chevalier, and Richard Brown, "The effects of grounding (earthing) on inflammation, the immune response, wound healing, and prevention and treatment of chronic inflammation and autoimmune diseases," *J Inflamm Res* 8 (March 24, 2015), 83–96.

40   Gaetan Chevalier et al, "Earthing: Health Implications of Reconnecting the Human Body to the Earth's Surface Electrons," *Journal of Environmental and Public Health* 12 (2012).

accumulated charge that we get from non-native and unnatural electromagnetic frequencies. As we are constantly exposing ourselves to Wi-Fi, cell phones, dirty electricity, and other frequencies that disrupt the natural flow of our own electrical makeup, we begin to acquire a charge inside our body that fills us with too many positive protons. This keeps us in a constant and chronic state of stress and inflammation. In short, the theory of grounding says that when we place our bare feet on the earth, we create a properly conductive relationship that is not disrupted by rubber. We can basically discharge what our bodies have accumulated into the earth.

Therefore, the simple solution is to cultivate ongoing awareness that this is a critical component of the healing pathways within our bodies. Awareness will lead to creating habits around the practice of grounding. This might mean walking barefoot in your backyard first thing in the morning and last thing at night. This might mean taking walks barefoot through a meadow or swimming in the ocean. Take every opportunity you can find throughout the day to ground yourself to the natural world and discharge that negative buildup. These habits can be extremely beneficial when we are traveling and we want to mitigate or dramatically diminish the negative effects of jet lag. Sunlight, good water, and earthing are three of the most powerful tools (and two of them are free!) that we can use to offset jet lag and inflammatory reactions in our body.

Technology is catching on to this practice too. There is a growing market for special pads, mats, mattresses, and other items made to be compatible with a properly grounded prong or outlet in your home. Proceed with caution, though, because if not properly grounded, these tools can create a worsening effect.

EMFs may be a new concept for you. If you're just learning about EMFs for the first time, it can be overwhelming and challenging to accept. Having studied health and wellness for many years now, I can tell you that this is a topic not to be taken lightly. I encourage you to do your own research and make educated decisions about your relationship to EMFs. Just do your best, seek out help if possible, and try to have an open mind about the presence and negative effects of EMFs. Our technology is evolving faster than ever, and the companies that profit aren't about to slow progress for the sake of human health. Don't expect companies to safeguard your health; take your well-being into your own hands under the guidance of a trusted health practitioner.

CHAPTER 9

ADDRESSING COVID NATURALLY

Were you wondering when we would talk about COVID-19? In the previous chapters, we've been laying the foundation for cultivating a holistic lifestyle, which is the most powerful thing you can do to safeguard your health.

The human body is an incredible biological symphony of cells, a microbiome (bacteria), and a virome (virus). These all need to work in a symbiotic way to provide us with health, vitality, and balance. So, that's step one—prioritize a holistic lifestyle. The beauty of shifting your focus to lifelong health is that it takes the fear out of the equation. You are taking back your power. You are the one in charge of ensuring your health. You're not waiting for a virus to victimize you.

So let's narrow our focus a bit. What are some specific things we can do to address COVID naturally? We can turn our attention to strengthening the immune system. Let's look at some nature-based elements to consider when improving and assisting your body's innate immune system.

The following recommendations come from many years of investigating the quality and integrity of the products. The alternative health market abounds with vitamins, herbs, powders, and supplements. Now more than ever, you need to be well educated and selective about what products you choose to integrate into your body. Be careful not to overdo it with supplements. However, the right supplements can be powerful tools to support the human body as it tries to adapt to a highly unnatural environment. Please note that the following recommendations are extremely well researched and highly specific. Please also remember that I am not a doctor and these recommendations are not meant to take the place of medical advice. Please do your own research and consult with a certified health professional.

Hormone D

In the alternative health world, vitamin D is being highlighted as a potential counter to COVID-19. Although there is some validity to this recommendation, we have to consider context as a key factor. Vitamin D is not really a vitamin; it's more of a steroid hormone. It is created naturally by our bodies via sunlight and cholesterol. The body absorbs UV light and converts wavelength ranges between 290 and 329 nm (nanometers) into natural hormone D. Most manufacturers and supplement designer fail to consider the full mechanism of how this works; nature's method is superior. Both plants and animals have the ability to create vitamin D from UV light—therefore, this nutrient is present in our foods in different forms. Most vitamin D supplements are isolated and supply unnatural single frequencies of D. This can oftentimes lead to toxic amounts and excess calcium buildup, leading to calcification.

Yes, hormone D is essential for immunity and is a valid support in light of the current situation. We should, however, try to manage the requirements by using sunlight and nutrient-dense foods. If someone lives in a northern latitude where sunlight is scarce, it's best to saturate storage reserves of vitamin D in the summer months. If this is not enough, then a UV light and red light therapy will typically suffice instead of introducing isolated chemical vitamin D supplements into the body.

Vitamin A

Chronic hypervitaminosis A, when a person has too much vitamin A in their body, is a factor that often gets missed. This usually arises from excessive amounts of isolated retinoic acid or synthetic and highly concentrated amounts of vitamin A. It usually accumulates in the liver over time and fails to be emptied out properly. This may be the product of a combination of GMO/glyphosate and pharmaceutical concentrates of retinoic acid (from things like Accutane or birth control) combined with excessive vitamin D supplementation or heavy use of topical vitamin D in sunscreen or beauty products. Sometimes excess vitamin A can result from ingesting abnormal doses of carotenoid-rich foods from excessive juicing or from drinking green smoothies. It can also come from over-supplementation with too much concentrated carotenoids like astaxanthin.

If you have challenges like eczema, autoimmune symptoms, G.I. distress, or blurred vision, then vitamin A toxicity is worth exploring. Check to see if you have been exposed to concentrated sources or supplements high in vitamin A for a period of time. By eliminating these sources and reducing foods high in carotenoids and vitamin A, these issues can actually be resolved. The liver will empty its accumulation and eventually return to normal metabolism.

Note: Be careful using herbs, especially if they are not adaptogenic or tonic. Adaptogenic or tonic herbs are usually safe to use daily, as they are not concentrated in specific constituents that throw body chemistry out of balance. They tend to modulate the immune system in the direction that it needs most help. Do your research and cycle herbs if using them in supplement form. The best approach to getting them in your diet in a balanced manner is by adding the raw form through cooking. Things like turmeric, ginger, garlic, cilantro, rosemary, oregano, and basil can be quite medicinal in small doses when used to flavor your food. If you're going to use herbs as supplements, just remember to let research, context, and intuition guide you.

Vitamin C

When we think of combatting flu, vitamin C easily comes to mind. However, the common approach is megadosing with ascorbic acid (the most active component of vitamin C). I recommend a different approach. When we start to put all the lifestyle pieces of the puzzle together, we stop thinking in terms of isolated vitamins and minerals. This is true with consumption of vitamin C. Instead of taking a vitamin C pill, I recommend eating a variety of berries, as well as lemons, oranges, and other citrus fruits. In cases where the body is under stress and the immune system is being challenged, there might be a need for extra vitamin C in supplement form. In that case, I recommend starting with a whole food blend of vitamin C (typically containing concentrated forms of acerola, camu, and/ or alma berries). These are not only safe and effective, but also offer a better complex of other biological constituents. I like North American Herb & Spice's Purely-C.[41]

You might also consider bee products like wild honey, bee pollen, and even royal jelly, which all have high levels of food-based C and B vitamins. Plus, the vast nutrient complexity of bee products is incredibly powerful for boosting immunity.

Understanding Key Minerals

After over eleven years of being active in the health field and working with hundreds of people, I can say without a doubt that everyone needs magnesium.

You know by now that I preach context and nuance, but because our soils are so depleted, our nutrition is less than optimal. So many factors come in to play here like genetically modified organisms, chemicals, pesticides, herbicides, and an altered hydrological cycle of the planet (acid rain). Add to that the chronic stress that is rampant in our modern

---

41   https://www.northamericanherbandspice.com/shop/purely-c/

world, and you have the perfect recipe for depleting magnesium levels in the body. For these reasons, I feel that everyone needs magnesium.

It is clear through testing and observation that most people (over 90%) in the United States are suffering from magnesium deficiencies. Even Mayo Clinic recognizes this reality. Not only is magnesium extremely important for over a few thousand enzyme and overall biochemical reactions in the body, it is also directly tied to levels of calcium in the body. Magnesium deficiency is usually accompanied by high levels of calcium buildup inside the body. This leads to a cascade of inflammatory reactions, deposit formation, fibrosis, and overall mitochondrial dysfunction (energy loss). All these affect the immune system and make us more susceptible to infections.

The most bioavailable and effective way to fix magnesium in the body is by using magnesium bicarbonate. Magnesium bicarbonate is the hydrated electrolyte salt that is made in the pancreas and the liver. It has always been naturally occurring in water. Magnesium bicarbonate not only has the ability to remedy the calcium magnesium ratio, but it's also quite effective in dissolving any stone formation and calcium deposits in the body. Magnesium in bicarbonate form also assists with the clearing of the voltage-gated calcium channels, which leads to more energy and better overall mitochondrial function. Magnesium bicarbonate as an electrolyte acts as a superconductor and therefore helps to improve the electrical potential of the body. It is also essential for the body to achieve pH balance.

Understanding your magnesium burn rate and the amount of magnesium you need for overall functioning is also essential. Most of us are depleting our magnesium stores or pushing this burn rate because of chronic stress due to financial, emotional, and other challenges that become a constant strain on our physiology. Nutritional deficiency and exposure to the wrong type of water or hard water, pollutants, and other environmental factors also lead to the depletion of magnesium stores in the body. Key elements in nutrition also play a role—think excess consumption of PUFA (polyunsaturated fatty acids) from vegetable oils like canola, soybean, margarine, sunflower, flax, and even omega-3 supplementation in the form of fish, krill, and algae oil; extreme dieting; and macronutrient and micronutrient deficiencies. Finally, the influence of electromagnetic frequencies is essential to understand when considering overall cell health and magnesium. EMFs can affect the magnesium burn rate and the amount of magnesium that gets depleted from the body. As you can see, it's extremely important that everyone get magnesium in the form of bicarbonate. We can also consider using magnesium in topical form or in baths to help build magnesium stores.

I recommend you get magnesium in bicarbonate form from Live Pristine.[42]

Iron Overload

The issue of iron is quite tricky. Some people are diagnosed with anemia and are encouraged to take iron supplements. However, I've often observed that this leads to worsening symptoms because the patient is misdiagnosed and is actually dealing with a deficiency in copper. Bioavailable copper is essential to creating new oxygenated blood, and when excess iron is present, copper is antagonized and displaced. Because of NPK farming, acid rain, fortification of iron, and excessive consumption of industrial type foods, most people today have excess levels or accumulation of iron. This creates a "rusting" effect inside the body. Removing concentrated forms of iron is essential to improving circulation. Again, using magnesium bicarbonate and increasing oxygenation with the principles in this book will help to resolve iron issues. Another way you can resolve iron overload is to donate blood. This can be done one to four times per year based on proper blood tests. This is one form of removing rust from the body.

---

42 https://livepristine.com/collections/electrolyte-balance

If you suspect you may have iron overload, it is best to test using the Mag-Zinc-Copper Panel.[43]

It would be wise to discuss your results with a practitioner who understands the role of iron, copper, magnesium, and vitamins A and D.

Copper not Zinc

Although most people, even health experts, are recommending you take zinc to guard against COVID, I recommend you proceed with caution when considering zinc supplementation. Testing blood for this marker is important, as you don't want to displace other minerals by overloading zinc. Most people have either faulty copper metabolism or a deficiency of copper. Copper and zinc are antagonists; when there is iron excess, which also affects copper, then zinc will most likely be out of balance. So, test for zinc in your blood, and you may find that a concentrated supplement won't be necessary. The best option to improve overall copper will be to include liver in your diet once or twice a week, depending on your specific needs. If this isn't practical or possible then using a desiccated liver supplement can be helpful—again, do your research and consult a health expert. If you decide to go forward with a supplement, I recommend the Grass Fed Beef Liver[44] from Ancestral Supplements.

Nature-Based Anti-inflammatories and Immune Boosters

Consider the following natural supplements to aid as anti-inflammatories and immune boosters.

Turmeric

Turmeric root is one of the most wonderful spices to incorporate into your diet. The active component curcumin is known to be an

---

43   https://requestatest.com/mag-zinc-copper-panel-with-iron-panel-plus-vitamin-a-and-vitamin-d-test

44   https://ancestralsupplements.com/desiccated-liver

anti-inflammatory and has incredible properties to improve cellular function. Use it in soups and golden milk.

Ginger

Ginger is also extremely beneficial for circulation and improving oxygenation of blood. As such, it keeps the immune system supported. Ginger has a high ability to capture light photons, is extremely beneficial for gut health, and acts as a powerful overall tonic for the body.

Pomegranate and tart cherry

A great deal of literature has shown the benefits of pomegranate and tart cherry as heart and circulatory system optimizers. The blood-like red color of these two fruits comes from an antioxidant factor that assists with cellular and epithelial integrity.

Bee products

Wild raw honey, bee pollen, royal jelly (if available), and propolis[45] are all extremely beneficial to overall health. These are not only some of the top antioxidant foods around, but they're also the best food-based supplements for B vitamins. Having proper levels of B vitamins is essential for calcium and overall metabolism. These are all good sources of vitamin C as well.

Medicinal Mushrooms

The adaptogenic or immune modulating effects of medicinal mushrooms are not to be underestimated. These immune enhancing medicinal foods are not only safe, but they also offer constituents that are normally not found in standard diets. Medicinal mushrooms are also tailor-made to support our bodies when there is excessive pollution and/or a high viral (exosome) load. Some of the most common and

---

45   A mixture of propolis and honey is extremely powerful as a natural antibiotic, antiseptic, and overall immunity booster.

powerful medicinal mushrooms are cordyceps, chaga, reishi, turkey tail, lion's mane, and agaricus. If you're looking for a reliable source, I recommend Alpha Dynamics[46] and Surthrival.[47]

Near-Infrared and Red Light Therapy

You read in an early chapter about the harmful effects of blue light. The excess amount of artificial blue light has shifted our natural rhythms and brought forth an epidemic of sleep disturbances, hormonal dysfunction, and a host of other mitochondrial-based challenges. As with any challenge, there's always a solution. Red light or light emitted in the frequencies between 650 to 850nm is the antidote to blue light dominance—especially at night.

Near-infrared light is the key frequency that penetrates deep inside our bodies to affect mitochondrial and cell function. Red light therapy has been shown to improve ATP function, reduce reactive oxygen species, and oxygenate the body. All these factors help build natural immunity as well. Red light also enhances collagen integrity, which in turn assists with skin health. It helps open the detox pathways and assists the liver and kidneys in decongesting action. It also helps with muscle and joint pain, speeds up wound healing, and helps reduce stress.

The study of photobiomodulation, or the use of red and near-infrared light to positively affect health, is extensive and boasts a massive research base showing its benefits. In short, it's a non-thermal way of stimulating cells to produce more energy and reduce inflammation and pain. Devices, light panels, and even near-infrared bulbs present us with a powerful tool that will eventually become a necessary element in most people's homes. Sunlight, which emits all light frequencies, has historically been used as a therapeutic agent to heal skin conditions, autoimmune issues, and hormonal and digestive challenges.

---

46   https://alphadynamicshealth.com/?aff=19

47   https://www.surthrival.com/collections/medicinal-mushrooms-1

Moreover, low-level lasers that emit a more precise red light have also been successfully used for wound healing and ailments such as arthritis, carpal tunnel, and even fibromyalgia.

Today we see incredible growth in the use of LED red light devices in clinics, centers, and at home. My go-to red light tool, which I also use as a portable and in-house infrared sauna solution, is SaunaSpace.[48]

If you're looking for another option that is more concentrated-LED based, consider GembaRed[49] and EMR-TEK.[50] They are both small, family-based companies of high integrity.

When it comes to fighting COVID, we have to start by shifting our paradigm. We're talking about improving immunity and optimizing health for the long term. I've arrived at this position through many years of research, experimentation, and successful application on myself, friends, family, and clients. It represents probably one of the most sophisticated, advanced, and effective approaches to creating the most robust health. As we've said before: start small and build one habit at a time. Explore how to optimize your diet and consider how near-infrared and red light therapy can help you get healthy and stay healthy so you can face our post-COVID world without fear.

---

48   https://sauna.space/?rfsn=3334503.503b021eb
49   https://gembared.com
50   https://emr-tek.com

CHAPTER 10

CALCIFICATION, FIBROSIS, AND YELLOW FAT

The topic of this chapter is somewhat controversial. I invite you to approach it with an open mind. Popular messages about omega-3 fatty acids, calcification, and fibrosis abound. In this chapter, we'll examine an alternative message.

There are some key pillars most people miss when it comes to regenerative health. It's rare to find these principles anywhere else in the field. A good portion of these ideas I credit to the work of Glen Caulkins from Pristine Wellness in Laguna Beach. You've heard me talk about Glen before. His level of experience, knowledge, and consistent results make him stand out from the crowd. I would like to also acknowledge the work of Matt Blackburn. Matt has over twelve years of research and development in the field of health and wellness. Like me, Matt never stops learning and adapts his knowledge and practice based on the best and most current findings and research. Even though some of his views on social media may seem controversial, his work always aims to help people.

I highlight the work of Caulkins and Blackburn in the spirit of collaboration and gratitude. The more we spread the essential application of these alternative ideas, the faster we can progress as a species.

Degeneration, autoimmune challenges, hardening and stiffness of muscles throughout the body, and the little-known aspect of yellow fat accumulation are the top drivers of premature aging and overall failure of the human organism. In the following pages, I aim to make you aware of three key areas: calcification, fibrosis, and yellow fat disease. It's time that we create a roadmap to slow and prevent these challenges.

Calcification Defined

Calcium is a highly studied mineral in biochemistry. Most people relate calcium to having strong bones. Although in simple terms this is correct, there is a lot more to consider before we can get the whole story on calcium.

Unabsorbed calcium can lodge anywhere in our body. For instance, if it lodges in your bones and joints, it mimics arthritis; if it lodges in your heart, it mimics arterial lesions. Calcification or calcium poisoning can manifest as heart disease, cancer, wrinkled skin, kidney stones, osteoporosis, dental problems, bone spurs, cataracts and many other health problems.[51]

What are some of the unexplored factors that can lead to calcification? Maintaining the proper ratio between magnesium and calcium is critical to preventing soft tissue calcium deposits in the body. Chronic stress and inflammation lead to magnesium deficiency, which in turn affects the body's ability to metabolize calcium.

Exposure to and toxicity from unnatural substances can trigger this response. Acid rain and agro chemicals such as glyphosate (Roundup), other herbicides, pesticides, and chemical-laced non-organic food are key triggers of this accumulation of calcium deposits. Acid rain leads to a chronic rusting of the planet, delivered through its waterways, which leads to excess iron. Added to an excess accumulation of phosphorus and potassium from conventional non-organic foods, this leads to excess calcium in the cells.

Another potential toxic element that is rarely taken into consideration and that has a potential compounding effect on calcium is

---

51   Dr. Sircus, "Calcification and Its Treatment with Magnesium and Sodium Thiosulfate," December 8, 2009, https://drsircus.com/magnesium/calcification-and -its-treatment-with-magnesium-and-sodium-thiosulfate/.

the accumulation of synthetic vitamin A. Research is demonstrating that excess amounts of vitamin A accumulation in the liver can lead to autoimmune conditions. Although vitamin A has typically been observed as a beneficial fat-soluble vitamin, the way we fortify our processed foods with vitamin A can lead to overload of the wrong type for those whose diets rely heavily on these fortified foods. Synthetic supplementation, supernatural consumption of carotenoid-rich foods (think excess vegetable juicing), topical application via the skin, and a history of pharmaceutical-based products (e.g., Accutane) can also contribute to vitamin A overload. These can all cause gut irritation, which contributes to excessive calcium accumulation.

Due to the mainstream narrative that we're calcium deficient, many people supplement with synthetic and excessive amounts of actual calcium. Moreover, fortification of calcium and synthetic vitamin D in processed and prepackaged foods adds fuel to the fire.

Another possible cause of calcification is protein deficiency—more specifically, improper amino acid absorption and utilization. Although adequate protein consumption may seem inconsequential in a world where calories and food abound, there is a definite trend of dieting and consuming nutrient-deficient foods that inhibit protein synthesis. The prevalence of overly restrictive or extreme diets means many people are protein deficient, which affects their ability to metabolize calcium. Think excessive fasting and extreme low-calorie diets in the pursuit of weight loss. Many fad diets exclude macronutrients and whole food groups for long periods of time, causing chronic protein (amino acid) deficiency. This is especially evident in diets that restrict carbohydrates. Carbohydrates, often touted as a nonessential macronutrient, are actually essential for healthy metabolism; they're the body's primary and most effective fuel. Protein tends to be best absorbed when paired with some form of natural carbohydrate.

Other nutritional deficiencies are also common, leaving the body missing key elements for functional mitochondria. With calcification, we often see vitamins E and K (two important fat-soluble vitamins) missing or in low quantities because of Western diets and mineral deficiency from depleted soil. These factors have to be considered because many modern dietary programs are based on concepts and ideas that result in nutrient depletion. This becomes problematic in the long term, especially if it becomes intergenerational.

The effects of electromagnetic frequencies coming from cell towers, Wi-Fi, cell phones, dirty electricity, and 5G also play a role. These frequencies, although invisible, affect cellular and mitochondrial (energy) function in the body, especially the voltage-gated calcium channels inside the cell—pathways for cell communication and electron exchange. EMFs often lead to a buildup that creates poor conductivity. Again, this leads to crystal formations and overcalcification.

Overconsumption of fish oil, algae oil, flax oil, and vitamin D supplements can contribute to overcalcification too. These oils can slowly lead to lipofuscin or yellow fat disease (premature aging), another major factor in regulating calcium levels.

I have had the opportunity to witness all these factors affecting calcification for many years. As a bodyworker who understands not only fascia but the mechanisms of fibrosis, scar tissue, and calcium depositing in the soft tissue, I have observed this phenomenon as a major challenge in almost all of my clients.

Finally, water is perhaps the most critical element of the whole calcification story. Water that is used for drinking, cooking, making coffee, tea, etc. should be pristine and free of contaminants and industrial-based acids. There are many factors involved here, but hard water with high dissolved solids equals calcification. Please refer to chapter 4 for more information about how to prioritize clean drinking water.

What Is Fibrosis?

In simple terms, fibrosis is when scar tissue (also a form of calcification) builds up in excess throughout the body. This occurs mainly because around age twenty-seven we begin to produce fewer enzymes. This, in turn, begins a cascade of scar tissue buildup, thicker blood, immune dysregulation, aches, pains, and initial onset of arthritic symptoms. If this fibrosis does not stop and new enzymes are not created, starting around age forty-five we can start to see the lowering of sex hormones. This affects overall drive, mental ability, bone integrity, muscle mass, and constant stable energy. As this progresses, it can lead to nutrient deficiencies, mineral loss, and eventual organ failure.

Here's how classical naturopath and exercise physiologist Dr. William Wong explains the condition:

> Fibrosis can be found in many forms. In women it can manifest as the estrogen driven diseases of Fibrocystic Breast Disease, Uterine Fibroids, Endometriosis and Ovarian Cysts. It can also be found post operatively in the Lymphedema had after mastectomy as the fibrin clogs the lymphatic drainage channels and thickens the lymphatic fluid. In both sexes fibrosis forms the postoperative scar tissue that binds the intestines, or restricts the range of motion of a limb and joint or forms thickened scars and keloids marring cosmetic surgery. Fibrosis can develop in the arteries and forms the framework around which arterial sclerotic plaque builds. In COPD, Emphysema, Asthmatic and Chronic Bronchitis patients, fibrosis creates scar tissue as a spider web inside the lungs, restricting their expansion and clogging alveolar sacs to prevent O2 transfer to the blood. In men fibrosis grows inside the micro blood supply and spongy tissues of the penis, restricting blood flow and full expansion during erection. This is the main reason why erection size diminishes with age.[52]

---

52   Dr. William Wong ND, PhD, "Fibrosis: The Enemy of Life," Dr. Wong's Message, accessed November 30, 2020, https://drwongsmessage.com/fibrosis-enemy.

One of the main reasons this occurs is because of the slowing down of enzyme production. Most vitamins and minerals (which are really cofactors dependent on enzymes) do not work or get absorbed properly. This happens with amino acids as well. Excess estrogen from plastics and phytoestrogens from foods like soy and flax can worsen fibrosis as well as leading to depression, anxiety, weight gain, mood swings, loss of libido, and lowered immune function.

Solutions

So, what can we do about this? Consider the following and decide which of these might be the best step for you to integrate first.

1. Reduce stress and inflammation in general by better self-care, recovery, and rest. Practicing mindfulness and breath control, and improving sleep can help.

2. Reduce excess estrogen by eliminating plastics in food and water and reducing high-estrogen foods in your diet. The main ones to steer clear of are soy, flax, factory farm meat and poultry (these are usually pumped with hormones), and vegetable oils.

3. Help eliminate fibrosis through bodywork. Revisit the previous chapter on bodywork for specific recommendations.

4. Replenish enzyme stores. In a pristine environment, eating raw fruits and vegetables would be the go-to solution for adding more natural enzymes into the body. Unfortunately, because of chemicals, glyphosate, NPK farming, and acid rain, this has become a challenging approach. I'd caution against the popular practice of vegetable juicing. It would have been an effective strategy to increase enzymes in the past, but the solids (NPK) and pollutants from the produce make this approach counterproductive. A high-quality and effective systemic enzyme

product is a must-have product for today's circumstances. I like MitoLife's Dissolve-It-All[53] and Dr. Wong's Zymessence.[54]

5. Use magnesium. Again, everyone today needs magnesium. It is involved in almost all biological processes and reduces stress and fibrosis.

Finally, LivePristine's ANTIDOTE[55] is loaded with living enzymes. This is definitely one of the most-preferred ways to replenish enzyme stores in the body.

PUFAs and Yellow Fat Disease: A Silent Culprit

When I begin work with a new client, we typically start with an oil (ex)change. This is perhaps the most important change you can make in your kitchen. It has been shown to have one of the most profound impacts on improving overall health.

So what do I mean by an oil change?

Marketing and misguided nutritional information have sold most people in our society on the idea that heart-healthy oils come from plants. Actually, the exact opposite is true. For much of our evolution and prior to the Industrial Revolution, we used stable fat that doesn't oxidize and is heat resistant. These fats are primarily saturated and also monounsaturated (like olive oil). They come from sources like tallow, coconut, grass-fed butter, and ghee. The stable bond in saturated fat makes it more heat stable and safer, as it's less prone to oxidation. Lipid peroxidation (degradation of fat) occurs most in longer chain fatty acids found in PUFAs (polyunsaturated fatty acids) and even more so in HUFAs (highly unsaturated fatty acids). These come from vegetable

---

53   https://www.mitolife.co/collections/mitolife-products/products/dissolv-it-all ?variant=32895783698535

54   https://drwongsessentials.com/zymessence/

55   https://livepristine.com/products/antidote-the-ideal-superfood

oils that are very unstable and prone to rancidity and oxidation due to the number of double bonds found in their makeup.

The mainstream and even alternative health channels have led us to believe omega-3s are essential, "heart healthy," and beneficial. Omega-3s, however, like DHA (six double bonds), EPA (five double bonds), ALA (three double bonds), and linoleic acid (two double bonds) are unstable and oxidize very rapidly. These are found mainly in fish oil, algae oil, krill oil, flax oil, seeds, nuts, and some beans, grains, and legumes. If consumed from time to time in their whole food state, they are not as damaging, especially when accompanied by natural vitamin E (e.g., in almonds). When we consume oils like these and other PUFAs such as canola (rapeseed) oil, soybean oil, cottonseed oil, margarine, and other vegetable oils for consumption, we create a constant and chronic inflammatory state. This eventually leads to hormonal imbalance, gut issues, and calcification. When we pair this with mineral imbalances and iron overload (mainly from fortified foods, copper deficiency, NPK farming, and chemicals) we run into major health issues like heart disease, diabetes, mood and mental health disorders, Alzheimer's, premature aging, and even cancer. This can lead to a little-known condition called yellow fat disease or lipofuscin. This condition is unaddressed by most people and unacknowledged by most health professionals. It's a silent condition where the liver creates yellow fat or a nonalcoholic fatty liver condition. It also leads to interference with normal cell metabolism and opens up the possibility of cancer-promoting metabolic pathways. It vastly interferes with proper circulation and oxygenation of tissues. This is basically, as Atom Bergstrom, a leading researcher in yellow fat disease says, "death by a thousand paper cuts,"[56] and a major factor of rapid aging.

Unfortunately, we store PUFA in our fat. When you combine stress (high cortisol), EMF, roller-coaster dieting, dehydration, overtraining,

---

56   Atom Bergstrom, "Lipo-Gate/Omega-3 Watergate," One Radio Network, https://oneradionetwork.com/atoms-blog-articles/lipo-gate-omega-3-watergate/

and insufficient recovery, these stored PUFAs are released from fat into our bloodstream, creating improper metabolism and fibrosis, which can also lead to calcification and hardening of the arteries.

Our body temperature is 98.6. If we use this as the environment housing these PUFAs, then we can see, as an example, that it doesn't matter that our "healthy" flax oil was refrigerated in dark bottles. It will still oxidize and create inflammation inside our bodies.

Solutions

1. Rethink or stop supplementing with HUFAs: these are fish oil, algae oil, flax oil, and krill oil.

2. Whenever possible, avoid all PUFAs and hydrogenated oils in your diet: canola, soy, cottonseed, sunflower, peanut, safflower.

3. Switch to saturated fat as staples: grass-fed tallow, grass-fed butter/ghee, coconut oil, and the right and correctly raised lard (if you're okay with pork products).

4. Limit PUFA-containing foods in your diet. For example, don't eat beans every day. Do not consume too much trail mix or granola, often touted as a super "healthy" food. Excess consumption of peanut, seed, and nut butters also comes into play here.

5. Monounsaturated fats are good. It's great to incorporate organic first cold-pressed extra virgin olive oil.

6. Switch your protein powder. Pea and hemp not only have higher levels of phytoestrogen, but they are also a source of PUFA. It's best to switch to gelatin, collagen, and/or low-temperature grass-fed whole whey.

Supplements That Make a Difference

Some of the supplements you read about in chapter 9 you'll see repeated here. In the context of this chapter, they relate specifically to guarding against calcification, fibrosis, and yellow fat disease.

The supplement industry has been one of the fastest growing areas in the health and fitness industry for many years. As with anything, it has its benefits but also its downsides. The downside is not widely known and, therefore, is worth mentioning here. First of all, the supplement industry is highly unregulated. Second, people are confused about what they should and shouldn't be taking, so they're experimenting without context and without understanding the powerful effects some of these substances have on their biochemistry. If used incorrectly and under the wrong circumstances, supplements can become toxic and counterproductive. Humans are always looking for a magic pill; we should be very suspicious of any product that claims to solve all our problems.

In this section I want to highlight a few of the major supplements and food concentrates that often get people in trouble.

Before we dive in, it's important to note that anytime you want to start a supplement or herbal regimen, it's best to consult a qualified health professional who is well versed in the subject. Your gut sense and intuition are also worthy sources of innate guidance.

First, what to avoid:

- **Multivitamins.** These are typically low-quality and synthetic-based. Even if they're natural, they most likely have ingredients you don't need. This can lead to excess in the body and can create displacement or deficiencies of other vitamins and minerals.

- **Calcium.** Calcium without magnesium leads to calcification. An excess of this mineral creates soft tissue crystals, cement-like bodies, and arterial-circulatory blockages. It is extremely rare that someone actually needs a calcium supplement.

- **Omega-3 oil supplements.** Because of the way these contribute to yellow fat disease, I advise avoiding fish oil, algae, krill, flax, and all omega-3 supplements. Please refer back to the previous section on PUFAs and yellow fat for full details on why I don't recommend these.

What to include:

Remember to factor in context as you decide whether you're a good candidate for taking the following supplements. When taking part in any supplementation program, it's always best to do your own research. It's also very helpful to have guidance from a natural-minded and licensed health professional. In most cases, when using the following safe products, I typically suggest relying on the product recommendations for usage.

Be aware, though, that there are also individual circumstances that require fine-tuning these recommendations or even abstaining from using certain products. For example, consider Dr. Wong's writing about enzymes:

> Don't use the product if you are a hemophiliac or are on prescription blood thinners like Coumadin, Heparin and Plavix, without direct medical supervision. The enzymes cause the drugs to work better so there is the possibility of thinning the blood too much.[57]

- **Magnesium.** Again, almost everyone is deficient in magnesium today. Magnesium bicarbonate is my top choice, followed by topical magnesium chloride, and in some cases a high-quality blend of magnesium L-threonate, magnesium taurate, and magnesium glycinate.

---

57   William Wong ND, PhD, "What Are Systemic Enzymes and What Do They Do?" Ann Arbor Holistic Health, https://annarborholistichealth.com/2015-4-29-what-are-systemic-enzymes-and-what-do-they-do/.

- **Shilajit.** Throughout my years trying many supplements based upon testing and intuition, shilajit and magnesium are still my foundational products of choice. It is called the destroyer of weakness for good reason. Shilajit not only supplies the eighty-four organic minerals that are missing in the soil, but it also provides the highly important fulvic, humic, and ulmic acids as well. These weak organic acids are essential to keeping our ecosystems vibrant and helping the natural process of detoxification. I use and recommend shilajit from LivePristine and MitoLife.

- **Bee products.** The combination of a wild raw honey, bee pollen, royal jelly, and propolis is extremely beneficial to overall health. These are not only some of the top antioxidant foods around, but they are the best food-based supplements for B vitamins. Having proper levels of B vitamins is essential for immunity and overall metabolism.

- **Vitamins E and K2.** These two fat-soluble vitamins are deficient in our modern diets. Most people don't get enough, and these nutrients are necessary for many bodily functions. These are also key players in reducing calcium deposits, reducing excess estrogen and PUFA damage, and building high immunity. Again, I recommend MitoLife as a safe source.

Systemic Enzymes

Now that you know the factors that negatively affect calcification and metabolism, I want to share the benefits of systemic enzymes as a powerful and safe tool to reduce fibrosis and thus overall calcification.

You might have heard about digestive enzymes, which help break down food and protein. Some people might need these enzymes from time to time. Systemic enzymes, however, are used apart from food to lyse or eat up scar tissue. As I wrote earlier, fibrosis is a buildup in the body that often interferes with overall wellness and can lead to arthritic symptoms, mobility issues, chronic pain, and premature aging. The pancreas usually loses its ability to create endogenous enzymes after age twenty-seven, which can lead to estrogen dominance, ongoing inflammation, and calcification.

When we introduce systemic enzymes, they act almost like PAC-MAN, eating away at the crystals in fibrosis. In this way, we assist the body to turn back the clock and improve vitality and quality of life.

As one of the top enzyme researchers in the world, Dr. Wong writes about the many incredible benefits of systemic enzymes. He teaches how systemic enzymes help modulate the immune system and help clean blood. They are anti-inflammatory and anti-fibrosis; they even assist in fighting viruses. Consider this excerpt from an article on his website:

> Enzymes eat scar tissue and fibrosis. (7). Fibrosis is scar tissue and most doctors learn in anatomy that it is fibrosis that eventually kills us all. Let me explain. As we age, which starts at 27, we have a diminishing of the bodies' output of enzymes. This is because we make a finite amount of enzymes in a lifetime and we use up a good deal of them by the time we are 27. At that point, the body knows that if it keeps up that rate of consumption we'll run out of enzymes and be dead by the time we reach our 40s. (Cystic Fibrosis patients who have virtually no enzyme production to speak of, even as children, usually don't make it past their 20s before they die of the restriction and shrinkage in the lungs from the formation of fibrosis or scar tissue).
>
> So our body in its wisdom begins to dole out our enzymes with an eyedropper instead of with a tablespoon; as a result the repair mechanism of the body goes out of balance and has nothing to reduce the overabundance of fibrin it deposits in nearly everything from simple cuts, to the inside of our internal organs and blood

vessels. This is when most women begin to develop things like fibrocystic breast disease, uterine fibroids, endometriosis, and we all grow arterial sclerotic (meaning scar tissue) plaque, and have fibrin beginning to spider web its way inside of our internal organs, reducing their size and function over time. This is why as we age our wounds heal with thicker, less pliable, weaker and very visible scars. If we replace the lost enzymes we can control and reduce the amount of scar tissue and fibrosis our bodies have. As physicians in the US are now discovering, even old scar tissue can be "eaten away" from surgical wounds, pulmonary fibrosis, kidney fibrosis and even keloids years after their formation. Medical doctors in Europe and Asia have known this and have used orally administered enzymes for these situations for over 40 years![58]

I use two enzyme products myself and highly recommend them to others: MitoLife's Dissolve-It-All[59] and Dr. Wong's Zymessence.[60]

Medicinal Mushrooms

We discussed medicinal mushrooms earlier, but they're worth repeating in this specific context. Medicinal mushrooms are quite powerful and safe for enhancing immunity. They are considered adaptogen food/herbs in that they modulate the immune system toward a state of balance. They are very effective in enhancing whole body function, relieving stress, improving vitality, and boosting strength. I incorporate these as a staple in my diet through elixirs, smoothies, teas, and/or capsules.

Check out Alpha Dynamics[61] and Surthrival[62] for products.

---

58   William Wong ND, PhD, "What Are Systemic Enzymes and What Do They Do?"

59   https://www.mitolife.co/products/dissolv-it-all?variant=32895783698535

60   https://drwongsessentials.com/zymessence/

61   https://alphadynamicshealth.com/?aff=19

62   https://www.surthrival.com/collections/medicinal-mushrooms-1

Immunity over Vaccine

The topic of vaccines is always charged and prone to controversy. Mainstream medicine argues that vaccines benefit humankind, while alternative medicine takes a different view. Many people who argue against vaccinating have come to that stance because of adverse reactions they've witnessed in their children or themselves. They also see that pharmaceutical companies have a vested interest in the massive profits to be gained from potential sales, which is why they spearhead most of the research behind vaccination. There is plenty of valid and scientific information demonstrating that the concept of vaccination should be considered with more caution than the mainstream narrative provides.

No matter what you believe about vaccines, two things remain constant:

1. Humans were created with a vital and capable natural immune system. It's effective in regulating and adapting.

2. To this day there has never been a vaccine that has been proven to be safe and effective, and that has been placed through the proper trials. Most trials are funded by pharmaceutical companies, meaning the doctors and researchers taking part in the studies have financial ties to the companies making these products. In 2008, CBS reported on these questionable practices, reporting that:

The vaccine industry gives millions to the Academy of Pediatrics for conferences, grants, medical education classes, and even helped build their headquarters. The totals are kept secret, but public documents reveal bits and pieces.
A $342,000 payment from Wyeth, maker of the pneumococcal vaccine – which makes $2 billion a year in sales.
A $433,000 contribution from Merck, the same year the academy

endorsed Merck's HPV vaccine – which made $1.5 billion a year in sales.

Another top donor: Sanofi Aventis, maker of 17 vaccines and a new five-in-one combo shot just added to the childhood vaccine schedule last month.

Every Child By Two, a group that promotes early immunization for all children, admits the group takes money from the vaccine industry, too – but wouldn't tell us how much.[63]

The number of vaccines proven safe is zero;[64] the number of vaccines proven to be effective is zero, and the number of studies comparing children vaccinated with CDC schedule versus unvaccinated children is zero. I also recommend you explore the extensive fact sheet about vaccines compiled by the Weston A. Price Foundation.[65] It has a bulleted list of comprehensive vaccine information, followed by referenced studies and links.

From the perspective of rewilding, it's hard to make a case for vaccinations. An untested and potentially dangerous cocktail of unnatural and concentrated ingredients injected into the bloodstream is not in alignment with a rewilding approach. This bypasses all the body's natural self-defense mechanisms. Furthermore, it introduces foreign and potentially toxic materials in a forced manner.

In the context of COVID, the practice becomes even more questionable. The time line given to discover, produce, and distribute a

---

63   Sharyl Attkisson, "How Independent Are Vaccine Defenders," CBS News, June 25, 2008, https://www.cbsnews.com/news/how-independent-are-vaccine-defenders/.

64   Financial bias in this industry has led to widespread misinformation that fails to prove that vaccines were responsible for eradicating disease. I challenge you to conduct your own research of the current literature for conclusive proof of the safety and efficacy of vaccines. In many cases, it can be argued that hygiene, sanitation, and environmental improvement may have been contributing factors to phasing out the diseases.

65   https://www.westonaprice.org/wp-content/uploads/ImportantFacts.pdf

vaccine makes it nearly impossible to trust that it is safe. Moreover, if studies on previous coronaviruses in animals are any indication, the outlook isn't very promising. In fact, there is speculation that the animal trials for a COVID-19 vaccine have been skipped precisely because researchers already have enough data to show this is a dangerous avenue to explore on humans.

Finally, if a COVID vaccine produced similar outcomes to those of flu vaccines, then we already know they won't yield results.[66] Most of the time, flu vaccines make matters worse. Because the issue of vaccines is so polarized, I encourage you to do your own research and due diligence in order to make the most informed and best choices for yourself and your children.

It's vital that you question the efficacy and safety of vaccines for yourself. Learn about the massive profits made by the pharmaceutical industry that fund vaccine research. Pay attention to the trends on social and mass media where alternative channels and viewpoints are being censored. Consider my perspective that natural immunity is our best bet to overcome any health challenge—including COVID-19. It is paramount to understand that we have all the tools available for us to become healthy. The principles presented here in this book are designed to empower you to become highly adaptable to an ever-changing environment.

---

66   Much like the flu, COVID-19 tends to have ongoing mutations, which creates challenges to the efficacy of a vaccine. The vaccine may be outdated by the time the current flu or coronavirus season comes around.

CHAPTER 11

REWILD YOUR MIND, REWILD YOUR FREEDOM

Thus far, we've focused almost entirely on the health of the body. But if we are to maintain sovereignty over our lives, we cannot overlook the value of a sound mind. Rewilding your minds starts with self-love, acceptance, and self-awareness. Rewilding your mind also means holding a sense of respect for others. An open mind is a wild mind in a world changing as rapidly as ours is, allowing us to adapt to evolving circumstances.

Practicing awareness around what we do and how we think is a simple tool that often gets forgotten. Build habits into your lifestyle that constantly remind you to mind your own thoughts, feelings, and emotions. This will ultimately lead to true freedom.

We also need to talk about conformity. We must learn to get out of our comfort zones. It is healthy to question everything, especially when it relates to COVID-19.

Ask yourself:

- Where am I getting my news and current information?
- What biases and motivations are influencing this content?
- Are they financially and/or politically motivated?

Having a wild mind means that we face ourselves and take responsibility for the world around us. We hold the keys to our freedom. We all have the courage required to act; we are powerful beyond belief.

Since the beginning of the alleged pandemic, COVID has flipped our world on its head. Fear is at the root of this transformation. The news and nonstop social media reporting have waged an all-out assault on our minds. And yet, we have months of real-world experience inspiring doubt about the official story. It's enough to make you question everything. There is a subtle yet pervasive sense that something is not quite right. At times, that sense grows louder—when we hear of riots, financial pressures, lockdowns, mask mandates, and the like. Those who don't believe the mainstream narrative see how easily rights can be suppressed, the masses can be influenced, and political control can be exerted.

They say truth is stranger than fiction. The events of 2020 may be the best illustration of this truth. I wish these events were simply works of fiction, but the truth is that we are potentially facing a major mind control experiment. We have been desensitized through movies and TV shows to accept violence, extreme sexualization, and even child abuse. Our complacency has made this possible. We have accepted influences that have the potential to alter the way we think. Influences such as fluoride in water, chemicals, excess estrogen that disrupts hormone function, excessive dopamine affecting brain chemistry via technology, and algorithms in social media. It is time to rewild your mind. Snap out of the hypnotic state you've been conditioned to and take back your mental freedom.

Despite the fact that the COVID phenomenon has caused mental stagnation for so many, there is also a massive awakening happening. We can align with this awakening by becoming freethinking, conscientious humans. Together we can walk an evolutionary path toward peace and freedom.

Finally, this time in our history hands us an opportunity to become more spiritually minded. Faith in a higher power, your connection to God or the creating force of the universe is calling you to flourish into your innate goodness.

Here are some habits and lifestyle practices to consider to rewild your mind:

- Turn off notifications. This may seem like a trivial point, but the excessive rings, beeps, and flashes coming from notifications on our phones and computers have created a major Pavlovian effect, creating unnatural and excessive dopamine reactions in the brain. Go into your settings and turn off notifications.

- Intentionally limit your social media activity. It will save you time and will limit any false sense of reality plaguing your mind. The compulsive checking of social media can often lead to chronic sadness and a sense of not being enough. We compare our lives to people we don't even know. Social media posts exist without a wider context that is necessary to make meaning in real and lasting ways.

- Exercise your brain. Just like our muscles need a form of stimulus for growth, our brains require the same influence. Stick to puzzles, thinking games, chess, or other activities that challenge you.

- Remember to use red light as much as possible in the evenings to avoid exposure to artificial blue light at the wrong times; it affects your mood and thinking capacity. If you use an e-reader or tablet, get an orange or red light filter sheet on top to block the blue or green light. You can also set apps like Iris to change the settings on your monitor. All these changes also enhance your sleep, which will nourish your brain.

- Drink clean water. Remember the details presented in chapter 4. Elements like fluoride and xenoestrogens in water can definitely affect proper brain function and lead to unclear thinking and vulnerability to mental influence.

- Turn to nature. Give your brain a rest by stepping away from your devices. The best way to do that is to take a break and reconnect with nature. This includes walking on the beach, swimming in the ocean, going for a hike, and going camping. Even visiting a local park and leaving the phone in the car can sometimes be sufficient. These practices may seem minor, but they are essential to stabilizing brain waves. As an added bonus, remember to take off your shoes and ground wherever possible.

- Seek out alternative media sources in order to challenge the status quo. This is essential to your growth; this is how you get out of your comfort zone. Here are some that I like:
  - For information on COVID-19: Questioning COVID[67]
  - For social, political, economic, and health: One Radio Network,[68] Green Med Info,[69] Weston A. Price Foundation[70]
  - Other social, political, and philosophical channels: CRROW777 Radio[71]
  - The Corbett Report[72] on YouTube

Also, two great documentaries that highlight the effects and influence of big tech companies on our minds and choice are *The Social Dilemma* on Netflix and *The Creepy Line* on Amazon.

Our minds are malleable. We can decide which direction we want to take in life. Fear has long been utilized to influence our thoughts and choices. Now more than ever, it is crucial that we create habits and set systems that will protect our minds from being infiltrated. Now is the time to rewild your mind.

---

67 questioningcovid.com

68 oneradionetwork.com

69 https://www.greenmedinfo.com

70 https://www.westonaprice.org

71 https://www.crrow777radio.com

72 https://www.youtube.com/playlist?list=PLyY3zMxlwfECdyx8E-TmoBvryfrFx d55X

CHAPTER 12

HUNT, FORAGE, AND GROW
YOUR OWN FOOD

I hope you've noticed that I haven't argued for going back in time to a fully ancestral way of living. We can't ever truly go back. But we can acknowledge that we are more disconnected from our environment than ever before. We have to return to the truth that we are natural beings belonging to living symbiotic ecosystems. The practices of hunting, foraging, and growing our own food give us the opportunity to interact with nature in a way that is more dynamic and participatory.

Most of us have grown up in cities, where we're distanced from our food supply chain. Life post-COVID offers us the opportunity to get back to nature. This is essentially one of the most impactful ways we can rewild COVID.

Gardening

Start by creating a practice of hunting, gathering/foraging, and growing your own food. This might seem like an unattainable goal, but beginning is the first step in making remarkable changes. My family started by building a raised bed in our backyard. Growing edible plants and herbs doesn't require too much effort. You can use a little soil, a few seeds, and a few pots and start with some common herbs like basil that grow well indoors. Learning some simple sprouting techniques goes a long way to expanding seedlings like broccoli sprouts in a mason jar. These have a lot of micronutrients that add an excellent additional component to our other foundational foods.

With a little research you can find someone local who can help you begin a raised bed project in your front or back yard to get a few more calorie-dense foods coming with little effort. For instance, growing potatoes or sweet potatoes is as easy as cutting a few buds from an already cut potato and putting them into a coffee bag with leftover grounds. You can find these in your local coffee shop. For help getting started with your grow-at-home journey, check out the following resources:

- The Grow Network[73]
- Homesteading[74]
- Attainable Sustainable[75]

Foraging

We are also using awareness to obtain a better understanding of what's available in our local environment. In our case, we have wild fruit and coconuts available that we can forage in South Florida. Knowing some basic principles of foraging and learning more about your specific environment can lead you to places surprisingly abundant with food. In this area it's usually best to find a field guide or someone who has experience with foraging specific to where you live. A few good resources to get you started with foraging are:

- Arthur Haines[76]
- Forager's Harvest[77]
- Backyard Forager[78]

---

73   https://thegrownetwork.com/grow-half/

74   https://homesteading.com/homestead-handbook-grow-all-the-food-you-need-in-your-backyard/

75   https://www.attainable-sustainable.net/grow-your-own-food/

76   http://www.arthurhaines.com

77   https://www.foragersharvest.com/#/

78   https://www.backyardforager.com

- Edible Wild Food[79]

I'm a big fan of the work of Daniel Vitalis and his recent venture called WildFed.[80] This is an excellent place to begin if you're ready to incorporate the ideals of hunting and foraging into your lifestyle. Early in his career, Daniel embarked on a journey to discover what humans were meant to eat. He initially created a unique educational offering related to similar concepts on rewilding and exploring taboos that humans have avoided in a way that is limiting our progress as a species.

Daniel cultivated a successful public speaking career, an ethical and high-quality supplement line called Surthrival,[81] and an extremely successful podcast called Rewild Yourself.[82] After this, he decided to shift into a more hands-on approach as a modern-day hunter-gatherer with the purpose of putting his principles into practice. This has developed into a fantastic TV show and podcast called Wild Fed. These are two highly educational and entertaining resources. Find his wonderful show and podcast here:

https://www.wild-fed.com

Hunting

The next step is looking into invasive, conscious, and regenerative practices of hunting for food. In South Florida this is usually fishing, but it can also involve hunting invasive species of iguanas. Although I'm not there yet, I intend to integrate further into nature. Check out Back Country Hunters & Anglers[83] to get started.

---

79 https://www.ediblewildfood.com/foraging-for-food.aspx

80 https://www.wild-fed.com

81 https://www.surthrival.com

82 http://www.danielvitalis.com/rewild-yourself-podcast

83 https://www.backcountryhunters.org

Vote

Finally, don't forget to vote your values. Vote for regenerative farming, permaculture, and building self-sustainable communities. Visit Eat Wild,[84] a great website that provides a list of places and resources for more local and wild food. As we support these grassroots organizations and businesses, we're voting with our dollars. Together we can create the change we want to see in our world.

Find a mentor in whichever category is most interesting to you and choose a project to get started. Anything that moves you in the direction of achieving these lifestyle practices is a positive step forward.

---

84 http://eatwild.com

RELYING ON FAMILY, COMMUNITY, AND A GOOD SOUL

The goal of this book is to offer principles, tools, and strategies for total self-empowerment. And yet, we are not alone. Our culture promotes the idea that we have to pull ourselves out of adversity. But humans weren't made that way. We thrive in community; we long for social connection.

We have, for most of our evolution, relied on small egalitarian groups. In this way we survived and thrived in the wild. We all had roles and contributed to the greater good. I have hope that we can finally come together to recreate a modern version of this original design. Call this tribe, village life, small self-sustaining communities, or what have you, but this premise is essential for us to move into a "new normal" that we can be proud of. We need each other.

We can co-create networks, communities, and groups beyond our wildest imagination. The moment is now and the time is ours. Let's rewild COVID together and, better yet, let's rewild ourselves and together become a human family for the ages.

Thank you for reading this book. I hope it has given you perspective, inspiration, action steps, and avenues for further exploration. Please recommend this book and spread the word.

To your health and keep rewilding.

John

APPENDIXES

Appendix A: Cleaning Your Fridge, Pantry, and Beyond
Appendix B: Rotating Menu Ideas
Appendix C: Products, Supplements, and Health Investments
Appendix D: Mama Called the Doctor and the Doctor Said ...

CLEANING YOUR FRIDGE, PANTRY, AND BEYOND

Before we dive into the practical tools, I want to remind you to go step by step and set yourself up for success. Don't feel pressured to take on too much at once; if you feel overwhelmed, take it slow and make it simple. Understand that this is about making changes slowly over the long haul, and that means that results may not come immediately. Commit yourself to optimizing your health as a lifestyle and you'll set yourself up for success.

Marketing, food ad campaigns, and the extreme diet–minded culture have fed us messages about going all in and seeing dramatic results. Those kinds of messages are successful at selling a product but not at cultivating health for a lifetime.

A great place to start is cleaning out your kitchen. This will give you the highest benefit. An example of this is to recognize PUFAs in your diet and begin to eliminate those. These are mostly vegetable oils like canola, soybean, cottonseed, flaxseed, sunflower, and a few more (check out the lists at the end of this section). Another missed source of PUFAs is the excess amount of omega-3 oils like fish oil, krill, flax, and algae oils.

Next, build habits to avoid chemicals, especially glyphosate from wheat. This means buying organic at local markets whenever possible. The glyphosate effect is the main reason gluten-free has become popular. Do yourself a favor and go gluten-free; it's a great habit for weeding out glyphosate.

An important concept to help you on this journey of cleaning out your kitchen is to find replacements or alternatives for the items in your kitchen that are harder to part with. When you hit a roadblock, think alternatives.

Finally, make a new habit of reading labels to focus on ingredients. You might be used to prioritizing calories or carbs, but when you're building your kitchen for long-term health, it's first and foremost about nutrients. For instance, on a food label you see ingredients like: canola, soy, hydrogenated or partially hydrogenated oil, high fructose corn syrup, MSG, wheat, carrageenan, and the endless number of artificial and "natural" flavors that hardly anyone but a chemist can recognize. These are things to avoid from now on. You are looking for real foods, names you can pronounce and recognize as being living foods from the earth. Think fruits, vegetables, grass-fed beef, pasture-raised eggs and chicken, and wild-caught fish. These are all examples of healthy nutrient-dense foundational foods.

Now let's go over some of the key things to avoid and talk about what to substitute instead.

Avoid

- PUFAs (polyunsaturated fatty acids) in unnatural vegetable oils:
  - soy
  - canola (rapeseed)
  - corn
  - sunflower oils
  - margarine
  - cottonseed
  - vegan mayo
  - vegan butter and cheese
  - all other vegan substitutes

- HUFAs (highly unsaturated fatty acids):
  - fish oil
  - algae oil
  - krill oil
  - flaxseed oil
  - hemp seed oil
- soybeans
- corn syrup and high fructose corn syrup
- gluten and gluten-containing grains
  - wheat
  - barely
  - spelt
  - kamut
  - triticale
  - rye
- industrial/lab processed food—anything containing the above, plus:
  - artificial sweeteners
  - aspartame
  - MSG
  - chemicals
  - ingredient names that are difficult to pronounce
- fake plant protein food alternatives like Impossible Foods and Beyond Meat products
- factory farmed meats and eggs
- modern processed and conventionally raised meats with nitrites and nitrates:
  - salami

- ◦ ham
- ◦ jerky
- ◦ hot dogs
- ◦ sausages
- factory farmed homogenized, pasteurized milk
- farmed fish

Prioritize

- good fats and oils
  - ◦ coconut oil
  - ◦ first cold-pressed extra virgin olive oil (best consumed raw in salads and over cooked veggies)
  - ◦ grass-fed ghee and butter
  - ◦ grass-fed beef tallow
- protein sources and animal foods, best from wild or farm fresh (grass-fed) sources:
  - ◦ bison, elk, venison, grass-fed beef
  - ◦ farm fresh poultry—chicken, turkey, fresh eggs
  - ◦ wild fish and seafood[85]
  - ◦ other proteins (if tolerated)—soaked and sprouted legumes like lentils, mung beans, and garbanzo
- grain alternatives or pseudo "grains" (in moderation—best if soaked and sprouted)
  - ◦ buckwheat
  - ◦ quinoa

---

85   My recommendation is to limit these due to microplastics and contamination in the ocean. Once or twice a week these can be a natural source of zinc, selenium, and other minerals. It's always best to go for wild warmwater fish (lowest on PUFA), oysters, sardine, etc.

- ○ amaranth
- ○ wild rice
- ○ white basmati rice
- natural whole sugars (context is key)
  - ○ fruits—prioritize tropical fruits and berries; go easy on bananas
  - ○ wildflower raw honey
  - ○ coconut palm sugar
  - ○ maple syrup
  - ○ organic cane sugar
- dairy foods (if tolerated)
  - ○ grass-fed butter or ghee
  - ○ grass-fed whole whey protein
  - ○ grass-fed cultured yogurt
  - ○ kefir
  - ○ cheese (in moderation)
  - ○ grass-fed raw cow and goat milk (the lactose is mostly where people have issues here; enzymes in raw form should help, but always listen to your body)

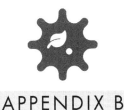

ROTATING MENU IDEAS

The following meal ideas and recipes are offered as guidance. These are time-tested, go-to food options that you can customize to suit your needs over time. Pay attention to the techniques at first; you can work with flavor and rotation as these changes become part of your lifestyle. Explore the catalogue of tutorials on rewildingcovid.com to learn more about what to eat, how to prepare meals, and how to navigate supermarkets and restaurants.

Rotating Menu Items

Red Meat Dishes

- Grass-fed beef kebabs with cauliflower mash and salad
- Bison burger in collard wrap or on chia seed "bread" with baked yucca fries and house greens
- Bison butternut chili
- Stuffed peppers with grass-fed turkey, cauliflower rice, carrots, and onion in tomato sauce
- Slow-cooked peach BBQ spare ribs
- Pumpkin beef burgers
- Grass-fed carne molida with cauliflower onion "rice" and steamed beets/carrots
- Grass-fed roast with mixed veggie stir-fry

- Grass-fed steak burrito in chia seed wrap with Mexican style salad
- Slow-cooked beef with purple potato, carrots, and broccoli
- Zucchini spaghetti with grass-fed meatballs, red sauce, and garlic squash plus house greens
- Grass-fed lamb and vegetable loaf with sautéed spinach and sweet potato mash
- Grass-fed liver/beef cubes and veggie medley with steamed yucca and salad
- Kale lamb burgers with cucumber noodles and cauliflower tabbouleh
- Lamb vegetable loaf

Farm Fresh Poultry

- Sunflower seed pesto artichoke chicken and veggies
- Sweet potato linguini, turkey meatballs with house greens
- Slow-cooked farm chicken leg and thigh with cauliflower and pea "rice"
- Ground turkey sandwich (collard wrap or chia seed "bread") with caramelized onions, olive oil mayo, and mustard with a side of purple fries and house greens
- Farm fresh chicken breast with buttered collard greens and avocado salsa
- Chicken veggie kebabs with cauliflower tabbouleh, side of no-bean hummus and kale chips
- Hearty vegetable chicken soup with real broth
- Stuffed portobello turkey caps with sweet potato fries and house greens
- Farm fresh chicken chop over curry cauliflower rice, with butternut cubes and sauerkraut

- Baked herb chicken over spaghetti squash and salad
- Honey mustard baked chicken thighs
- Pumpkin chicken chili with coleslaw
- Chicken cacciatore over "pasta"
- Turkey bacon apple stuffed chicken breasts
- Turkey bacon wrapped chicken breasts with tahini and sun-dried tomatoes
- Lemon Dijon grilled chicken with cauliflower mango "couscous"
- BBQ slow-cooked chicken
- Lemon garlic slow-cooked chicken
- Tomato basil slow-cooked chicken
- Butternut/carrot turkey loaf

Fish and Seafood

- Wild salmon nori wrap with kraut slaw and broccoli stir-fry
- Wild shrimp scampi with asparagus, radishes, yam noodles
- Wild scallop, sweet potato, and garlic linguini with root veggie salad
- Shrimp and vegetable cauliflower "fried rice" with hijiki salad
- Wild fish sticks with salad and baked yucca
- Untuna sardine casserole
- Haddock sprout rolls with seaweed salad and steamed carrots
- Wild garlic scallops with sautéed potato and collard greens
- Asparagus seafood crepe with plantain compote
- White sweet potato "pasta" with mushroom and shrimp
- Stuffed zucchini with crab pate and watercress pineapple salad
- Baked eggs with white fish and onion taro soup

Salads and Sides

- Steamed vegetables
- Sautéed vegetables
- Shaved radish, jicama, daikon medley
- Steamed yucca with ghee
- Sweet potato fries
- Sweet potato mash
- Cauliflower mash

Other

- Sweet potato vegetable frittata
- Sardine "tuna" salad with collard or chia seed wrap
- Vegetable egg omelet
- Vietnamese style spring rolls (has some rice flour)
- Sprouted lentil loaf with seasonal veggies
- Sprouted mung bean pesto "pasta" with cassava bread
- Sprouted lentil or mung bean vegetable medley with side
- Sprouted quinoa and veggies
- Soaked wild rice pilaf

PRODUCTS, SUPPLEMENTS, AND HEALTH INVESTMENTS

Throughout this book I have placed most of the focus on the importance of having a key foundation to achieving the best lifestyle possible. These principles have stood the test of time. However, we also live in a highly unnatural world with many challenges that stress our bodies. We face lots of deficient systems, many toxic elements, and depleted soils that lead to imbalances. Supplementation is a great way to start building a sustainable lifestyle. In this appendix, you'll find high-quality supplements I frequently recommend. These are the products I have found to provide the most benefit with the least amount of competing constituents, and that are the safest.

Products to Support Rewilding Your Lifestyle

- Live Pristine Water Solutions[86]
- Magnesium[87]
- Vitamin E, K, and Probiotic[88]
- Dr. Wong's Zymessence[89]
- MitoLife's Dissolve-It-All

---

86   https://livepristine.com/#

87   https://livepristine.com/collections/electrolyte-balance

88   https://www.mitolife.co/?afmc=2f&utm_campaign=2f&utm_source=leaddyno &utm_medium=affiliate

89   https://drwongsessentials.com/zymessence/ .

- LivePristine's Shilajit[90]
- MitoLife's Panacea[91]
- Surthrival's Colostrum Powder Products[92] for immune building
- Alpha Dynamic's medicinal mushrooms[93]
- Acumobility's bodywork tools[94]
- Sauna Space's infrared sauna[95]
- Blueshield EMF Scalar Wave Protection Technology[96]
- Testing for Iron, Copper, Zinc, and Magnesium[97]

Tools to Rewild Your Mind

- Questioning COVID[98]
- "Why Viruses Are Crucial to Life on this Planet, the Link Between Air Pollution, Glyphosate & Pandemics, Loss Of Biodiversity (& What We Can Do about It) & More with Dr. Zach Bush"[99]
- The Truth about Vitamin D[100]

---

90   https://livepristine.com/collections/pristinenutrition

91   https://www.mitolife.co/collections/mitolife-products/products/panacea?variant=32895787204711

92   https://www.surthrival.com/products/colostrum-powder?acc=47d1e990583c9c67424d369f3414728e

93   https://alphadynamicshealth.com/?aff=19

94   https://www.acumobility.com/?ref=61

95   https://sauna.space/?rfsn=3334503.503b021eb

96   https://www.blushield-us.com/?ref=84

97   https://requestatest.com/mag-zinc-copper-panel-with-iron-panel-testing

98   https://questioningcovid.com

99   https://bengreenfieldfitness.com/podcast/lifestyle-podcasts/glyphosate/

100   https://drive.google.com/file/d/0BweFjwhHC9atek9IV3ZzQk1Wamc/view?usp=sharing

- MitoLife Radio, "Why You Shouldn't Supplement Vitamin D with Jim Stephenson Jr and Morley Robbins"[101]
- Private Facebook group about research on vitamin D[102]

More about Glyphosate Toxicity in Humans

- "Glyphosate's Suppression of Cytochrome P450 Enzymes and Amino Acid Biosynthesis by the Gut Microbiome: Pathways to Modern Diseases" by Anthony Samsel and Stephanie Seneff[103]
- "Diminished brain resilience syndrome: A modern day neurological pathology of increased susceptibility to mild brain trauma, concussion, and downstream neurodegeneration" by Wendy A. Morley and Stephanie Seneff[104]
- "Elevated Serum Pesticide Levels and Risk for Alzheimer Disease" by Jason Richardson, PhD et al[105]

More on Yellow Fat Disease

- "Yellow Fat Disease is REAL & FISHY" by Atom Bergstrom[106]
- "Unsaturated Fatty Acids: Nutritionally Essential or Toxic?" by Ray Peat[107]
- "The Great Fish Oil Experiment" by Ray Peat[108]

---

101 https://podcasts.apple.com/us/podcast/mitolife-radio/id1454068609?i=100 0487452369

102 https://www.facebook.com/groups/517807781731760/

103 https://www.mdpi.com/1099-4300/15/4/1416

104 https://surgicalneurologyint.com/surgicalint-articles/diminished-brain-resili ence-syndrome-a-modern-day-neurological-pathology-of-increased-susceptibility -to-mild-brain-trauma-concussion-and-downstream-neurodegeneration

105 https://jamanetwork.com/article.aspx?articleid=1816015

106 http://www.solartiming.com/yellow-fat-disease-from-fish-oil-warning.php

107 http://raypeat.com/articles/articles/unsaturatedfats.shtml

108 http://raypeat.com/articles/articles/fishoil.shtml

- "Fats and Degeneration" by Ray Peat[109]

Vaccine Safety Education

- The Weston A. Price Foundation[110]
- Children's Health Defense[111]
- Green Med Info[112]
- Dr. Sherri Tenpenny[113]
- Vaxxter[114]
- Vactruth[115]
- Think Twice: Global Vaccine Institute[116]
- Project 180[117]

---

109   http://raypeat.com/articles/articles/fats-degeneration3.shtml
110   https://www.westonaprice.org/vaccinations/
111   https://childrenshealthdefense.org
112   https://www.greenmedinfo.com
113   https://www.drtenpenny.com
114   https://vaxxter.com
115   https://vactruth.com
116   http://thinktwice.com
117   https://www.goproject180.com/launch-page-1?affiliate_id=2005715

MAMA CALLED THE DOCTOR, AND THE DOCTOR SAID ...

The following is the best explanation of COVID-19 I've seen. The discussion is reproduced in its entirety with permission from the Ben Greenfield Podcast with special guest Zach Bush MD.[118]

．．．．．．．．．．．．．

And so, now, what we can look at, and this is what I've got in that HighWire,[119] I think we were able to show some of these on that. But my PowerPoint presentation on this, I can overlap those maps, and what you see is that it is Hubei Province is the overlap between the highest spraying in the world of glyphosate in concentration, as well as the highest antibiotic usage in pork production. And so, we have the most intense anti-microbial activity on the planet happening in Hubei. Coupled with the highest PM 2.5[120] in the world, as the pollution of Beijing pushes south from that city, it pushes right down into Hubei Province with the air pressure coming down from the north.

And so, we have this perfect opportunity to create a pandemic type relationship to a virus because we've created the pressure for shift through the herbicide, pesticide. So, we get all of this adaptation

---

[118] "Why Viruses Are Crucial to Life on This Planet, the Link between Air Pollution, Glyphosate & Pandemics, Loss of Biodiversity (& What We Can Do about It) & More with Dr. Zach Bush," Ben Greenfield Fitness, accessed December 3, 2020, https://bengreenfieldfitness.com/podcast/lifestyle-podcasts/glyphosate/.

[119] https://zachbushmd.com/video/the-highwire/

[120] https://www.health.ny.gov/environmental/indoors/air/pmq_a.htm

response from the genomics of both multicellular organisms, as well as bacteria and the like, and they're producing massive amounts of virus looking for adaptation advantages into the environment, then it binds to PM 2.5 and creates too much viral clumping in a very small particulate space. And then, that population has this lung that's going to absorb not just one virus, but could absorb dozens of viruses tied to one receptor into that body, into that single cell, and induce an overwhelm to those scissors that I described that are trying to keep us in balance with the viral intake, suddenly overwhelm the scissors. And simultaneous to that, if you have high glyphosate, the glyphosate is disrupting the very enzyme or the very proteins that would build the scissor system to clip it.

So, everywhere around the world, you're going to look for high glyphosate residues in the air and water system combined with high particulate matter of carbon in the atmosphere. And you know you're going to get high mortality from a virus that should have never caused any harm because it should have been in balance with us. And in fact, that's exactly what you see with coronavirus is the vast majority of people who are testing positive for coronavirus never got ill and/or had very minor symptoms. And so, the virus itself has no mortality. What has mortality is artificial chemical environments that are changing our relationship to this virus and inducing a toxic event. And it turns out that the toxic event, as mentioned at the very beginning of this description, was that these patients that are going to die from this condition aren't presenting with fever and elevated white blood cell count as if they're infected. They're actually presenting with hypoxia, a loss of oxygen-carrying capacity within the bloodstream.

When you get a hypoxic injury, the first things that happen is your lung will start to fill with fluid over the next few days from that hypoxic injury. At the same time, your entire body gets prone to blood clots from a deprivation of a number of proteins including like a HIF protein, which is a common one as a marker of hypoxia. And when HIF gets depleted, you'll go into this hypercoagulable state and you'll start causing microclots and go into multi-organ failure. What I just described is called histotoxic hypoxia.[121] It is not an infection, it's actually a poisoning of the bloodstream by many different toxins. But the most common one to cause histotoxic hypoxia happens to be cyanide. And cyanide happens to be at an extremely high rate of carry in PM 2.5.

So, now imagine, we've shown coronavirus tags onto PM 2.5, and actually so does influenza. And so, you get these viruses tagging. In the case of coronavirus, you can then tag ACE2 receptor[122] in the lung, you're going to absorb a high quantity of PM 2.5 tagged with cyanide into the bloodstream and cause hystotoxic hypoxia. And we're going to be told that that patient has an infection, so they're going to come in the hospital and we'll immediately treat them with antivirals and, bizarrely, antimicrobials like antiparasitics, like we were treating with the anti-malarial drug, hydroxychloroquine. We were treating with azithromycin, which is a common Z-Pak antibiotic. So, we're treating them as if they're infected, when in fact, they've had a poisoning of cyanide and other toxins within the PM 2.5 that's been carried in inadvertently by the virus. The virus itself causes no symptoms. Remember, the vast majority are asymptomatic or have very mild symptoms as they come into contact with some of the PM 2.5.

The final thing that we have to look at to really decode the whole pandemic event is, who was dying from it? What risk factors can we identify? Certainly, age was one of them, and it turns out that as we age, especially if we are in areas of high pollution, we will get minor changes within the lung consistent with chronic bronchitis or emphysema that upregulate the ACE2 receptor beyond its normal biologic function. So, these patients who are individuals that live in toxic environments (i.e., New York City, Northern Italy where we have high PM 2.5,

---

121   https://en.wikipedia.org/wiki/Histotoxic_hypoxia

122   https://en.wikipedia.org/wiki/Angiotensin-converting_enzyme_2

Ecuador, high mortality within some of the cities of Ecuador where we have very high PM 2.5). And basically, everywhere you look, Russia and otherwise, you're going to be looking for high PM 2.5 at chronic exposure rates and you're going to find that in inner city and high agricultural environments.

And so, the PM 2.5 goes up, cyanide goes up, and then the ACE2 receptor goes up based on this [00:50:39] _____ change. But it wasn't actually lung patients, ACE2 that were–I'm sorry, it wasn't actually lung patients that were showing the highest mortality from COVID, it was actually people with cardiovascular disease, diabetes, and kidney disease, which sounds like three very different disease processes until you consider the pharmacy that we have to put those patients on. As physicians, we know there's two drug classes that we have to put all three of those disease processes on, and that's an ACE inhibitor, which is a version of a blood pressure medicine, and a statin drug to control or reduce the cholesterol level produced by the liver.

And so, both ACE inhibitors and the statin drug happened to pharmaceutically increase the amount of ACE receptors in our lung and bloodstream and beyond. And so, fascinatingly, what we proved with this pandemic is that the pharmaceuticalization with ACE2 receptor increase combined with long-standing exposure to PM 2.5 and air pollution to upregulate these ACE2s combined with a virus that was just giving us an update, and the whole purpose of coronavirus—like all the other viruses—is to update the genome with the new adaptation process that is potentially life-giving to us. And we've seen this many times. If you get influenza, you're actually protected from many viruses if you get that genomic update.

And so, an important part of our genomic intelligence and our total immune system function relies on these genomic updates of viral syndromes. I'm very excited. I'm actually trying to put together a large multinational study right now looking at the long-term benefits of getting coronavirus. And I believe we're going to see less cancer, less autoimmune disease, and other things by people that went through that genetic update. And so, we're going to show those benefits over time. We can certainly show short-term benefits in other respiratory infections and stuff even within a year. Interestingly, we know that yet another risk factor for coronavirus and coronavirus mortality was influenza vaccination. It turns out that the influenza vaccine in 2017 in a military study in the U.S. was proven to increase the risk of six other respiratory viruses the following year, and one of those was coronavirus.

Zach: Precisely. That's great summary. Ultimately, we're dying from our own toxicity. Our toxicity is having all these downstream effects putting us in an artificial and disrupted relationship to the virum. Ten to the 31 viruses, if we lose our ability to be in balance with that, we will disappear very rapidly. And I believe that what we just saw, the amount of life that was lost, people died from complications of this virus again because the virus was carrying toxin and all this other stuff into the body. That was the tip of the iceberg. If we really did lose 200,000 people worldwide, that pales in comparison to the 250 million that we will lose over the next few years from just influenza.

We lose so many people to respiratory viruses every year and we pretend like it's the virus again and again that's causing this. And yet if you look at flu season as a whole, it only occurs during high environmental carbon exposure. This gets really interesting, actually. If you just google CO2 or greenhouse gas patterns in the atmosphere over the course of a year, by the time we hit September and October after a robust growing season in the northern hemisphere, there is almost no CO2 and methane left in the environment, and we've absorbed all of it through plant life and soil life pulling it down. There's only 4% of the 100% of the carbon that we produce over those months left in the atmosphere.

But then we go into fall and between November first and the third week of November, there's an explosion of CO2 and methane and other carbon particulate in the air as we go into fall. We suddenly lose that whole absorptive machinery of all the trees, and the greenery, and the soil. And then, we see in the third week of November, every single year, flu season starts, and we pretend like that's a virus causing that. It is absolutely biologically impossible that the third week of November every year sees a virus go pandemic. That's not what's happening. These viruses are ubiquitous all the time and yet our relationship to that virus suddenly changes every year in the third week of November because of the amount of carbon that we are producing that cannot be reabsorbed into that.

And so, the respiratory flu season is the result of huge amount of carbon, and the amount of it that's in the air by the time you hit March and April is insane. The whole northern hemisphere is bright red by satellite imaging there looking at CO_2 concentration. You can't even see the continents through the coloration of the maps. And so, we have this toxic stew by March and April, which is exactly when we saw the highest mortality from COVID. And then, by June, right in the second week of June, you see all of that disappear as the explosion of greenery happens across the northern hemisphere, and we reverse that pattern. And of course, as of June, we see this huge decrease globally of the amount of coronavirus.

You need to be careful about what you're hearing on the news. On the news, they say, "Oh, there's been a spike in number of cases of coronavirus." But if you look at the sheer number of daily cases in a "spike" right now, they are a fraction of what they were happening in April. And so, the total number of cases will keep going up because with time, more of us should be seeing this virus, we should go into a herd immunity, which doesn't mean that we're killing this virus, it means that we're now in a balanced genomic relationship to this virus over the next 12 to 18 months. We saw this with SARS, we saw this with MERS that within two years, there's no more of the virus causing any problem measurably anywhere in the world because the genomics of the population around the pockets where the virus occurred have developed that herd immunity.

And it's important that we realize that herd immunity doesn't need to be 94% of Americans or some 70% of Americans as we've been told by the CDC and stuff we need to vaccinate everybody so we can get to herd immunity. That's not how it works. Herd immunity only is necessary in the pockets where the virus is in high concentration in production and in binding to PM 2.5. So, really, all we need is 60% to 70% of the population having seen that virus in areas like New York City, Louisiana, Northern Italy. In those small pockets, we'll see that high concentration of exposure and then immune balance with that viral information, and then the syndrome will go away and nobody will ever die again of COVID. That's what happened with again SARS, MERS, which were two other coronaviruses nearly identical.

And so, we're spending literally billions of dollars to produce a vaccine for a virus that's going to be in a homeostasis balance within the next 12 months with our population. We don't need a vaccine to do that. Furthermore, we've tried to make RNA vaccines many, many times in the past, including with SARS and MERS, and we fail every time. RNA viruses are classically very disruptive to human biology and the immune system itself because it causes hyperreactivity. In fact, we saw just in the human study that just got put out, Dr. Fauci's company that he was invested in and all these billionaires invested in, they all jumped in on this one company that looked to be the most promising and they were the first to finish clinical trial in humans. And we saw a huge percentage of those developing this hyperreactivity capacity where they did fine with the vaccine. But if they see coronavirus next year, they are very likely to die from it because now they're hypersensitive to that stimulus.

And so, this has happened with RNA vaccine efforts over and over again. This one repeated it. And so, we have this ludicrous belief that viruses are bad for us, we have a ludicrous belief that our immune system relies on antibodies to prevent these infections, we have a ludicrous belief that vaccines are part of our balance with these things. So, we've just totally lost track of the last 30 years of science, just simply haven't impacted our current policy-making, drug development and the like. And that's not unusual. This isn't like a conspiracy theory. It actually consistently takes 20 to 30 years for new science to percolate into clinical care. And it doesn't matter if that's a breakthrough in science around cancer or immunity.

Zach: I think that we have to take a moment just to acknowledge the crisis we have right now around George Floyd's death. And it has ignited awareness on an extraordinary level, and this gives me again hope for the planet like we haven't paid attention to the death of the planet as we need to. We haven't changed. In the same way, for hundreds of years, we have subconsciously accepted the systemic and systematic suppression of black people within the United States. Slavery, of course, being the obvious one that marched on, but with the 13th Amendment, we re-enslaved black men in particular through the 13th Amendment when we said that we would take away their voting rights and all of their rights that we had given back to them after slavery if they were convicted of a crime. And so, through a loophole within the 13th Amendment, we created a re-enslavement of the black peoples within our country, and there has been systematic and systematic depreciation of their value and closing of doors very early in their life toward the opportunities that many other minorities even enjoy.

And so, I think that the lesson that we can take from this last hour of conversation around the microbiome is actually quite profound. The microbiome, meaning, the vast majority of life on Earth, bacteria, fungi, parasites, protozoa, archaea, this huge kingdom of single cellular and diverse life forms, five million species of fungi, 30,000 species of bacteria, 300,000 species of parasites, the numbers go on and on, then you get into 10 to the 31 viruses in the air. Life around us has evolved because of its capacity. And in fact, written into its code, the need and desire for biodiversity. If we were to align our socioeconomics and politics and social behavior to that natural law of nature, which is biodiversity and communication are the two most important features of health, what would our society look like if we did communication and saw biodiversity as the highest order of function of a society?

We would not recognize success or GDP unless it was measured by how biodiverse is your land and how biodiverse are your peoples. That would create a different world for us. Black Lives Matter is an interesting take on what we're seeing with viruses. Black Lives Matter is basically stating, "Here's the most suppressed black male demographic within your nation for hundreds of years." Pay attention here to your biggest mistake, your most grave misperception, and give back civil liberties and opportunity there. In the same way, we are going to need to adopt a virus, "The Viruses Matter" mindset. Viruses are our pathway to biodiversification just as the correction of our age-old, 200-year-old laws and legal structures, prison systems, police behavior. As soon as we change that behavior toward blacks, it will have an immediate ramification for Asians, Hispanics, women, children, all of the suppressed minorities. If we change our relationship in the same way to the viruses where we finally accept that these are not against us, they are actually for us, and we adopt a scientific and medical approach to embracing the viruses and finding a homeostasis balance with those viruses, it will inform a biodiversity where all the rest of the minorities within our mind, the bacteria, the fungi, and the rest will also enjoy new civil liberties within human biology.

And so, I think we see enormous opportunity to recognize that communication and biodiversity are the highest valuation on the planet, whether we look under a microscope or look across large socioeconomic systems. We have to embrace that biodiversity and we must do it in a fashion of speed of adoption, of transformation that has never been achieved before. We need a true metamorphosis, not change. Change isn't fast enough. We have proven again and again that we change slowly. We need a transformational mindset. We need a true metamorphosis of philosophy to realize that we are a very small piece of life on the planet, and we are only going to be valuable to this planet, and we will only be allowed to survive the next 70, 80 years if we find our role of biodiversity within us and around us.

ABOUT THE AUTHOR

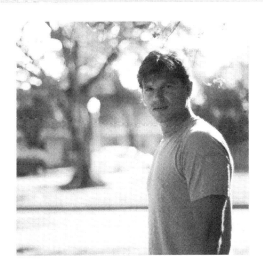

Establishing himself as one of South Florida's most groundbreaking and pioneering leaders in the health field, John Schott set himself apart from the pack early in his career with the opening of his restaurant and retail space, Lifefood Gourmet, South Florida's first gourmet health food restaurant. His food and health services have touched the lives of high-profile celebrities, athletes, and executives. He is also very mindful of the value of giving back and volunteers his time to various charitable causes, including implementing nutritional youth outreach programs and to teaching underprivileged children about healthy cooking and lifestyles.

John has studied closely with the top pioneering authors & practitioners for the last 14 years in the alternative health field. His knowledge of and experience with detoxification, nutritional cleansing, and wellness & lifestyle coaching is second to none. His practitioner model has been refined from a decade of apprenticeship, self-study, and hands-on application with hundreds of clients. John has in-depth insights into areas of health pertaining to nutritional timing (or "time conscious" eating), Gerson Therapy, and other alternative healing modalities & longevity strategies. He has created health and performance programs for some of the world's highest performance professionals and leads workshops and detox retreats in Florida and South America. John is the host of the *Rewild Humanity Podcast* and also offers a signature Rewild Humanity group coaching program online for ultimate health transformation.

Visit RewildingCovid.com to sign up for the latest news and natural health updates.

A SMALL FAVOR

Thanks so much for investing your time reading through this book. I hope that it has empowered you to take your wellness and immunity into your own hands and resist the forces leading us to ill health.

Please take just a moment to share your thoughts in a review wherever you purchased this book.

Readers rely on honest, thoughtful feedback from the wider community to help them make more informed decisions. It also helps me as an author refine my message and deliver relevant information and content my readers need.

I read each review personally and appreciate your honest feedback. Thanks again!

John